Dropping the Baby
and Other Scary Thoughts

Dropping the Baby

and Other Scary Thoughts

Breaking the Cycle of Unwanted
Thoughts in Motherhood

Karen Kleiman and Amy Wenzel

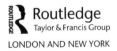
Routledge
Taylor & Francis Group

LONDON AND NEW YORK

Routledge
Taylor & Francis Group
711 Third Avenue
New York, NY 10017

Routledge
Taylor & Francis Group
2 Park Square, Milton Park, Abingdon,
Oxfordshire OX14 4RN

International Standard Book Number: 978-0-415-87700-8 (Hardback)

Library of Congress Cataloging-in-Publication Data

Kleiman, Karen R.
   Dropping the baby and other scary thoughts : breaking the cycle of unwanted thoughts in motherhood / by Karen Kleiman, Amy Wenzel.
     p. cm.
   Includes bibliographical references and index.
   ISBN 978-0-415-87700-8 (hardback : alk. paper)
   1. Postpartum depression. 2. Motherhood--Psychological aspects. 3. Childbirth--Psychological aspects. 4. Mothers--Mental health. I. Wenzel, Amy. II. Title.

RG850.K54 2010
618.7'6--dc22
                                              2010026696

ISBN 978-0-415-87700-8 (hbk)
ISBN 978-1-138-87271-4 (pbk)

This book is dedicated to Ilyene Barsky, MSW,

whose words, wisdom, and infinite presence continue

to inspire and heal postpartum women.

Contents

Preface ix
Foreword xiii
Acknowledgments xvii
The Authors xix

SECTION I   What's Going On

Chapter 1   A Mother's Anxiety.. 3

Chapter 2   A Closer Look... 21

Chapter 3   Why Am I Having Scary Thoughts?................................ 39

SECTION II   Clinical Concerns

Chapter 4   How Do You Know If You Need Help?............................ 59

Chapter 5   Barriers to Relief 79

Chapter 6   Screening for Scary Thoughts 97

SECTION III   Breaking the
Cycle of Scary Thoughts

Chapter 7   Things You Can Do to Feel Better 117

Chapter 8 Can You Really Change How You Think?..................... 143

Chapter 9 Professional Treatment Options.................................. 159

Chapter 10 How Others Can Help...................................... 177

Chapter 11 Your Personal Treatment Plan 191

Chapter 12 Living With Uncertainty 211

Afterword.. 221

References... 227

Index.. 237

Preface

You've just had a baby, and you're having thoughts that are scaring you. Thoughts that don't make sense. Thoughts about bad things happening to your baby by accident, by illness, or by your own actions. Maybe your thoughts are about harm coming to your partner or yourself. You wonder, *Why would I be thinking these things? Maybe I shouldn't have had this baby. Maybe something is wrong with my mind. Could I be going crazy?*

Your impulse is to run, to hide, and to deny that these thoughts are even there.

Motherhood and scary thoughts. To most, this is an oxymoron, a contradiction in terms. After all, if motherhood embodies the bliss that so many envision, how do we make sense out of the egregious thoughts that often present themselves during this time?

If you're reading this book because you or someone you love is struggling with distressing thoughts after having a baby, it is our hope that you will find comfort, explanations, and coping strategies to understand and manage this phenomenon better. Some of you may have been diagnosed with postpartum anxiety or depression; others may be wondering if one of these diagnoses might apply to them. The information in this book will be helpful whether or not you have been formally diagnosed with a postpartum anxiety or mood disorder. After all, having a baby and having scary thoughts are a disturbing combination, whether or not there is an associated diagnosis.

When we envisioned this book, we initially felt intimidated by three sets of challenges. The first was the taboo surrounding this phenomenon. Could we effectively and compassionately tackle a subject that is so taboo and so shocking—to consumers and healthcare professionals alike—that both groups frequently avoid addressing it altogether? Could our efforts cut through this resistance and misinformation in a meaningful way, while getting to the core of the pain? And would our efforts lead to more effective identification, referrals, and treatment when indicated, and, most importantly, greater understanding and comfort for the suffering mother? This was our clinical challenge.

Our second set of challenges rested with our audiences. In our clinical practices, we recognized a scarcity of accurate information on this topic for both women and the professionals who treat them. The vast experiences of a postpartum woman, whether at home with her baby, in her doctor's office, in a therapist's office, or discussing her leaking breasts with a neighbor, are profoundly intimate. With her tremendous bodily changes, her relationships, her expectations of perfection, her self-esteem, her sleep deprivation, her racing thoughts, and everything in between, everything suddenly feels up close and personal. Even under the best circumstances, when everyone is healthy and happy, unpredictable days are long, nights are longer, and adjustments are made on a minute-by-minute basis. All too often, the unique needs of a postpartum woman slip through the cracks of the medical and social community at large.

We have also found that a large number of postpartum women are surrounded by supportive friends, family, and healthcare practitioners who may not have accurate information regarding the symptoms of distress during this vulnerable time. In fact, many women come to our clinical practices after previously seeing one or more clinicians who, unfortunately, have misconstrued the circumstances and unwittingly exacerbated the anxiety.

Thus, we were struck by the concurrent need for both postpartum women and their healthcare providers to have access to accurate information. Could we effectively speak to both—the mother who is struggling and the healthcare professionals and therapists who are in a position to help her? One may be desperately trying to cope with terrible thoughts in her head, and the other is seeking state-of-the-art assessment techniques and treatment options, as well as the research to back them up. We concluded that because of the intimate nature of this work and the potential urgency for accurate information, the mothers and their providers could be served by the information in these pages.

The bottom line is that both mothers and providers are searching for and are in desperate need of this information. For this reason, we decided to speak to both simultaneously. At certain points in the book, it will be evident when our emphasis is directed to the mother or to the healthcare provider. However, it is our fervent belief that each can bring what has been learned into the other's realm. At the end of each chapter, we offer a summary in the form of a **Take-Home Point for Mothers** and a **Clinician Note.**

Our final set of challenges was the merging of our two very different voices. Karen would flippantly claim that she was the touchy-feely part of the book, or the enthusiastic writer, and that Amy was the academic, providing the conceptual framework. This may be true, but as it happens, Amy's robust academic and research background and Karen's extensive clinical experience created a perfect combination of energy and expertise for this delicate subject matter.

With these challenges carefully considered and sufficiently under control, we are confident that our readers will find the information and support that they need. In moving forward, readers will gain a deeper understanding of the phenomenon of unwanted thoughts during motherhood, including how common they are, why they occur, and what a mother can do about it.

HOW TO USE THIS BOOK

The tone of the book is geared toward you, the postpartum woman who may be struggling with scary thoughts, although it is important that healthcare professionals be aware of and integrate all the information into their practice with postpartum women. This book provides a much needed resource for mothers and clinicians who are forced to confront these negative thoughts by outlining the precise nature of these thoughts and how to manage them. These topics will be discussed within the context of motherhood, keeping in mind that some readers are not clinically anxious or depressed and that some are experiencing these troubling thoughts as symptoms of an anxiety or mood disorder. Having this information at hand will provide initial relief and help to normalize the experience, as well as augment recovery if a reader is in treatment for a postpartum anxiety or mood disorder.

This book is divided into three sections. Section I, *What's Going On,* contains definitions of various types of scary thoughts and provides a context for how common these thoughts really are. Section II, *Clinical Concerns,* explores the barriers to disclosing these thoughts and the screening and diagnostic implications for healthcare practitioners. In Section III, *Breaking the Cycle of Scary Thoughts,* we explore actions women can take immediately to feel better and continue to apply as they navigate their personal experience. Within this last section, in Chapter 11, we have included a personal treatment plan for the reader to keep a record of experiences and progress. Some women might find it helpful to check in with this chapter while they are starting the book and keep notes as they go along. Others might prefer to wait until they reach Chapter 11 and then put together a treatment plan after integrating what they have learned. Readers should rely on their personal styles and use this book in whatever manner is most helpful to them.

Readers should be careful to read the parts that pertain to them and be mindful of any triggers that may heighten their anxiety. It is not uncommon for books on distressing thoughts and emotions to aggravate anxiety to some extent, but we are hopeful that if they stick with it, readers will find the support they need to persevere until they achieve the relief they are seeking.

If, at any point along the way, you think that reading this book is making you feel worse, put it down. You might want someone you care about to read it and then discuss some of it with him or her. It is our hope, however, that you will be validated and reassured to read that what you are experiencing is a universal human condition that is not unique to the postpartum period, though it is definitely amplified during this time.

This is not easy work, and you should be commended for your effort to confront that which is frightening you. Even if your effort is completely driven by fear and you don't necessarily feel you deserve credit for confronting it, any energy you put forth toward acknowledging your experience and seeking support for it is indeed praiseworthy. Reading this book, along with your commitment to learn more about what is frightening you, is your first step toward reclaiming control in your life.

Karen Kleiman

Amy Wenzel

Foreword

From the moment my first baby was born, I fretted over him relentlessly. When I found out he had jaundice, a very common illness for newborns, I was convinced he was in mortal danger and refused to leave the hospital when I was discharged before he was. When we came home to the kind and experienced baby nurse that we had hired to guide me in the first week, I wouldn't allow her to do *anything* because I was sure my baby would think *she* was his mother and not me. (I sent her home, as I recall, on day 2 or 3.) I couldn't sleep when the baby slept because I felt I had to wash baby clothes and scrub bottles and make sure everything was ready when he awoke. Even at night, I couldn't go back to sleep after waking to feed him because my mind was filled with racing thoughts.

I was sure this was normal. After all, every new mother is worried, right? At first I believed that this must be what the transition to motherhood was like. I tried to pull myself together. I thought that perhaps if I got a little more time as a mom under my belt things might start looking up.

My lack of sleep, incessant worrying, and increasing inability to eat only made things tumble further downhill. I couldn't figure out why I was so anxious all the time. I felt helpless and unable to care for myself or my child. I started to become convinced that he would never love me. Then I hit the absolute depths of despair when, at around 7 or 8 weeks postpartum, I had my first intrusive thought: "What if I smothered him with the burp cloth?" There are no words to describe what it feels like to have such thoughts pop into your head. Needless to say, I was terrified. I continued having disturbing thoughts, like "What if I drowned him in the bathtub?" and "What if I dropped him down the stairs?" They plagued me throughout the day, each one crippling me more and more.

At the time I went through this, I had never heard of what authors Kleiman and Wenzel refer to as "scary thoughts." I didn't know it was possible for a normal, everyday person like me to have horrible notions come into her mind that she didn't want or instigate in any way. No one told me this was a temporary symptom and something that was fully treatable. I came to the only conclusion I could: I'd gone completely crazy, never to be the same again. I felt I was a terrible human being who had no business being a mother. What a difference it would have made had I known what was happening to me.

Because I understand exactly how devastating postpartum anxiety in all its forms can be, I am all the more honored to be able to introduce *Dropping the Baby and Other Scary Thoughts: Breaking the Cycle of Unwanted Thoughts in Motherhood.* Karen Kleiman is the queen of postpartum depression-related literature. I know no other way to say it. She has written everything from the seminal *This Isn't What I Expected: Overcoming Postpartum Depression* to *What Am I Thinking? Having a Baby After Postpartum Depression* to *The Postpartum Husband* and *Therapy and the Postpartum Woman.* I have every single one of her books in my library and I refer to them time and time again—both for my own writing and as referrals for the women who reach out to me needing support. Amy Wenzel has conducted much research on postpartum anxiety and has recently authored a book on anxiety disorders in pregnant and postpartum women. Readers can trust that what Kleiman and Wenzel write in *Dropping the Baby and Other Scary Thoughts* is the best information out there about how to get through debilitating anxiety and worry related to childbirth.

This book is sorely needed. More women than people realize are experiencing scary thoughts. Many of these women are having difficulty getting through even a single day of being a mother and are not functioning as they would like. Even in this day and age, when so many work hard to educate both women and healthcare providers about postpartum anxiety and depression, many women still have no idea what is wrong with them. Until I got help, I didn't know the first thing about what was happening to me. I didn't know that my illness had a name and that I could get better (see Chapter 2). I didn't know in what ways I may have been sabotaging my chance at recovery (see Chapter 5). I didn't know there were effective self-help methods that would augment the treatment I'd later receive (see Chapter 7).

I am in constant contact with women who don't get the same kind of expert help I did. Some have their worries dismissed as normal without further discussion. Others are told to wait it out and see what happens. Others are so afraid that they wouldn't dare tell someone what is wrong for fear of losing their children and being locked up forever. Some are even misdiagnosed as having postpartum psychosis and are unnecessarily hospitalized. None of these outcomes is acceptable.

Women who are suffering from excessive worry, scary thoughts, or panic attacks or who are concerned they may have postpartum depression, postpartum anxiety, or postpartum OCD now have the information they need at their fingertips. There is no other resource on this topic as comprehensive as *Dropping the Baby and Other Scary Thoughts*. The book tackles a taboo subject and carefully takes the reader through the stages of early identification of what scary thoughts are, understanding how common they are, and, perhaps most importantly, coming to terms with what is happening and what to do about it.

With their combined expertise and warmth, Kleiman and Wenzel present us with a much needed resource to help mothers in great distress feel comforted and hopeful. They are also careful to address the unique challenges of therapists and other healthcare providers who are in a position to support postpartum women. The information in this book is well researched, sensitively delivered, and essential for any mother struggling with thoughts that are scaring her.

Katherine Stone
Founder, Postpartum Progress

Acknowledgments

We are greatly indebted to all the women who have courageously shared their most private and painful thoughts. We sincerely hope that this book will comfort you.

Words cannot express our gratitude to Trish McGarrigle, who sat on Karen's living room floor night after night making sure every sentence said what we wanted it to say. Trish's steadfast commitment and outstanding editorial skills were an asset throughout this project.

A special thanks to our families, especially our husbands, Bruce and Tim, for their constant love and gracious acceptance of our devotion to this work. Amy would especially like to acknowledge her soon-to-be-born daughter, who was with her throughout the writing of this book and who provided many opportunities to practice the strategies to manage scary thoughts.

We are also extremely grateful to our publisher George Zimmar, project coordinator Marta Moldvai, and Karen's new best friend and editor Judith Simon, whose unwavering dedication to our work made it possible for us to offer these words of explanation and support to the women who have asked for them.

The Authors

Karen Kleiman, MSW, licensed clinical social worker, is founder and director of The Postpartum Stress Center. She is author of several books on postpartum depression, including *This Isn't What I Expected* (Bantam Books), and an internationally recognized postpartum depression expert. After graduating in 1980 from the University of Illinois at Chicago with her masters in social work, she began her practice as a psychotherapist, specializing in women's mental health issues. In 1988, she founded The Postpartum Stress Center, a treatment facility for prenatal and postpartum depression and a training center for therapists. In March 2009, she opened The Postpartum Stress & Family Wellness Center in New Jersey, expanding services to include the treatment of children and adolescents.

In addition to her clinical practice, Karen teaches a specialized postgraduate course for clinicians and provides training programs for healthcare professionals and mentoring opportunities for therapists who wish to specialize in the treatment of perinatal mood and anxiety disorders. Her work has been featured in local and national magazines, numerous radio shows, and local and national television shows, including *Inside Edition, The Oprah Winfrey Show,* and *NBC Nightly News with Tom Brokaw.* She is frequently asked to consult and lecture on the topic of postpartum mood and anxiety disorders. Karen lives with her family outside Philadelphia, Pennsylvania.

Amy Wenzel received her PhD in clinical psychology from the University of Iowa, followed by her clinical psychology internship at the University of Wisconsin Medical School. She has served on the faculties of the University of Pennsylvania School of Medicine, the American College of Norway, and the University of North Dakota. Her research has been funded by the National Institutes of Mental Health, the American Foundation for Suicide Prevention, and the National Alliance for Research on Schizophrenia and Depression. She is author of *Anxiety Disorders in Childbearing Women: Diagnosis and Treatment* (APA Books) and editor of the forthcoming *Handbook of Perinatal Psychology* (Oxford University Press), as well as author or editor of books on topics such as cognitive therapy, cognitive research methods, and close relationships.

Her areas of research and clinical expertise are in perinatal anxiety disorders, interpersonal functioning in anxiety disorders, suicide prevention, and cognitive therapy; she has published more than 75 articles and chapters on these topics. She lectures nationally on issues relevant to mental health and psychotherapy and provides ongoing supervision to clinical psychologists, social workers, and psychiatric nurses. She currently divides her time among scholarly research, training and consultation, and clinical practice.

Section I

What's Going On

1

A Mother's Anxiety

I'm just going to check once more to make sure she's breathing.

Watch his head, hold his head!

Be careful, don't drop the baby!

New mothers take their mothering seriously. The awesome responsibility of caring for a newborn naturally warrants a heightened sense of vigilance. Sometimes this necessary state of watchfulness can be confusing. At every turn, a new mother believes a crisis is looming. Afraid of slipping and dropping the baby, she holds him extra tightly while she goes down the stairs. Afraid of a disaster in the night, she keeps herself awake to hear the silent sounds of breathing. If she falls asleep from sheer fatigue, she dreams of causing the baby harm through her own negligence.

One woman described visions of watching her 1-week-old son tumble out of her arms, landing head first onto the ceramic tile at the base of the stairs. Each time she was at the top of the stairs, upon taking the first step, she would gaze at what seemed like an eternity of winding stairs fading into oblivion. The flight of steps seemed to trigger a perpetual loop of recurring anxiety. No matter how careful she was, no matter how many times she safely reached the bottom, she reported that this image entered her mind every time she walked painstakingly down the steps. Every single time.

It's hard being a mother. Even under the best of circumstances. Mothers know this. Fathers know this. Society knows this. People who have never had children know this. It's hard caring so much, working relentlessly, feeling emotions that are unfamiliar and intense. It's hard being a mother whether one feels healthy and strong or whether one is encumbered by symptoms of anxiety or depression.

This slippery slope of distress is a risk for the population at large, but it is particularly menacing for women who are emotionally vulnerable following childbirth. A woman who is experiencing significant postpartum anxiety and depression knows this only too well. Trying hard to make sense of the recent emotional upheaval, she resorts to her own misguided interpretation of her feelings. She may worry about her varying symptoms and why they are there in the first place. She wonders if she is overprotecting her child by checking on him through the night or if this is just what mothers who love their babies do. She obsesses, quite diligently, about every detail of every thought and every feeling.

The mood of a woman experiencing such thoughts can alternate from euphoria to hopelessness in the blink of an eye. Her thoughts can range from deciding that having a baby was the best decision in her life to wondering if her baby would be better off with another mother. She might express her love for her baby with awe-inspiring and enduring affection, or she might hope that if she just wished hard enough, her baby would simply go away. A mother's wish to be the best mother she can be is difficult to reconcile with the simultaneous wish for her baby, or herself, to disappear forever. A large majority of postpartum women battle these contradictions with fierce determination and tireless resolve, but eventually each one will grow weary. Very weary.

The period following the birth of a child is a transitional time that can challenge a woman in profound ways. She is deprived of precious sleep, she is hormonally compromised, and sometimes she is thinking things she cannot believe are crossing her mind. If a new mother experiences thoughts that are uncomfortable to her during a time when her family, friends, and society expect her to feel blissful, she is likely to be overcome by guilt and a crushing sense of failure.

In spite of advances in public awareness of postpartum depression and anxiety disorders and increased attention to the experience of motherhood on the whole, expectations that new mothers feel good about themselves—and particularly about their babies—remain extremely high. Happy mothers = good mothers. This view continues to be a driving principle within a culture that claims to have the best interests of both mother and baby at heart. But until we recognize and accept the very real fact that being a mother doesn't always feel so good, we continue to corner mothers into the untenable position of pretending that everything is fine.

This prevailing notion that mothers should endlessly radiate joy paradoxically keeps them feeling sick longer.

AREN'T ALL NEW MOTHERS ANXIOUS?

Yes. Experts and mothers equally agree, with no reservations, that all new mothers experience anxiety. It can manifest as a physical symptom (*My heart drops when my baby cries*) or a behavioral response (*I have to double-check to make sure the baby is breathing*). It can also impact the way a person thinks (*I hope the baby is okay. I probably shouldn't have brought him out to the store; now he's probably going to get sick*). All of these, as well as other manifestations, are normal responses to the stressors of motherhood.

Historically, anxiety is understood to be an ally of sorts; it is an internal signal that can serve to protect us, motivate us, and alert us to danger. Anxiety is a natural response to threatening triggers. In this way, anxiety reactions are understood to be adaptive and, to a large extent, primal and instinctive. When people experience a dangerous or threatening situation, the fight-or-flight response is activated. This survival response pumps adrenaline throughout the body, setting off a surge of physical changes, including rapid heart rate, palpitations, and increased blood pressure. The purpose of this response is to prepare us for action. Most of us can recall a time in our lives when we responded this way, either to a very real threat or to a situation that we perceived as threatening to our health or well-being.

There are also times when anxiety leads to productive changes. In these cases, one might worry for a short time before engaging in some behavior that effectively lessens the worry and may impact the outcome in a positive way. If, for instance, a mother worried that her hand-me-down car seat wasn't safe enough for her new baby, she might decide to purchase a new one, thereby virtually eliminating the worry. Some might claim this is how one "worries well." In these instances, the initial worry prompts a response that favorably changes the outcome and lessens the anxiety.

Many women reading this book might think that sounds good on paper, but when it comes to the perceived well-being of their own babies, it's an entirely different matter. Exploring the concept of anxiety within the context of motherhood can stir up emotions that range from discomfort to madness. Mothers seem to wonder endlessly whether their own emotions are normal or whether they are overreacting. Depending on personalities and predispositions, some women tend to think it's everyone else who is overreacting and that their own instincts and imaginings are right on target; others lean toward self-deprecating responses and presume they must always be mistaken. Emotions can be so erratic during this time that it's hard for a mother to discern what is within normal limits and what is not.

When we take a closer look into the restless mind of a new mother, we find an array of anxious responses that generally fall into three categories along a continuum. At one end, there is the *all-new-mothers-feel-that-way* truism with which many women reassure themselves—for example, *I wonder if she's getting enough milk.* These are anxieties that fit comfortably within a socially acceptable definition of "new-mother anxiety." At the other end, there is the *something-must-be-wrong-with-me* state of being that causes substantial distress—for instance, *I cannot leave the house until the baby is 6 months old. I heard that before they are 6 months old they are susceptible to megagerms that can cause fatal diseases. I've tried to leave, but I can't breathe when I go outside; my chest starts pounding, and tears pour out of my eyes. It's just not worth it.* Such thoughts represent anxieties that interfere with functioning and require professional attention. Lastly, by far the most common scenario—*Is this normal for me to feel this way?*—is made up of those anxieties that teeter between the two ends of the continuum.

The majority of women who seek professional support for symptoms of postpartum anxiety and depression are ones who find themselves wavering between the two extremes: *Is what I am thinking normal?* and *Could I be going crazy?* They know they are far more anxious than they've ever been before and wonder how much is too much anxiety? They worry that they are way too nervous, hypervigilant, or obsessive—so much some days that they fear they might really be going mad. Thus, if we view these responses along a continuum, with "normal" anxiety at one end and severe, incapacitating anxiety at the other end, the preponderance of postpartum women who struggle with symptoms of anxiety fall somewhere between the two points, leaving a great deal of room for doubt and uncertainty.

It stands to reason that motherhood and anxiety would go hand in hand. However, the unpredictable nature of the role combines with anxiety in combustible fashion, leaving many women feeling vulnerable and unprepared. Nearly everyone, including the new mother, her loved ones, and healthcare providers, expects some degree of anxiety to go with this territory. But this is the crux of the problem. It is often difficult to distinguish "normal" anxiety from that which may be a symptom of an anxiety disorder or an expression of postpartum depression. Most are not surprised or terribly concerned when the mother of a 1-week-old infant reports that she is nervous about her baby's well-being, worried that he's not eating enough, or wondering if he's going to die from SIDS if she doesn't go check on him throughout the night.

Because this natural response to protect the newborn is often expressed with hyperalertness, another part of the problem is that healthcare providers, more often than not, dismiss early expressions of anxiety as par for the course. The intrinsic and primal nature of a mother's anxiety can unfortunately lead to a false sense of complacency in healthcare providers. In addition, in spite of the current academic and legislative focus on postpartum depression and anxiety disorders, the emphasis remains on depressive symptoms. Women remain reluctant to express anxiety partly because it can feel so "whiny" or irrelevant. A woman's urgent desire for relief is too often construed as neediness, a label that serves no purpose to a weakening spirit. Regrettably, many doctors reinforce this notion by referring to anxiety as merely a nuisance for the postpartum woman: something she just needs to get used to. But, at its worst, anxiety can be crippling; within this context of the postpartum period, it can be an important signal that requires further attention.

Who decides what's "normal"? To be sure, tolerance levels vary from one woman to another. What feels acceptable to one may feel unbearable to another. Postpartum women can sustain considerable levels of worry and nervousness. It seems to be an occupational hazard, part of the maternal instinct to protect, nurture, hover, and worry. When we listen to what women are saying about their anxiety, we hear them using descriptions such as, *I'm having a nervous breakdown. I'm a nervous wreck. I'm a worrywart. I'm nuts. I'm sick with worry. I'm freaking out. I'm losing my mind.* And then, of course, there's the patronizing voice from well-meaning healthcare providers or family members who don't quite understand such as, *Oh, it's nothing* and *It's just anxiety.* In this chapter, we explore some of the many characteristics that comprise anxious thinking patterns in order to validate some of the thoughts with which you may be struggling.

SCARY THOUGHTS

Scary thoughts is the expression we use in this book to encompass any and all categories of upsetting thinking that can interfere with the well-being of a new mother. Scary thoughts refer to negative, repetitive, unwanted, and/or intrusive thoughts or images that can bombard you at any time. We gave the use of this term considerable thought after initial reservation from esteemed colleagues who wondered whether the phrase might minimize the gravity of the subject matter. There was concern that "scary thoughts" might conjure up cartoon-like images of a child's nightmare that would be unsuitable for the clinical seriousness of the experience, such as monsters under the bed. But monsters are indeed terrifying. They are gigantic, nasty beasts who are ugly and gross and scary. And yet, there is no real danger. There is only perceived peril. And this is precisely the point.

Scary thoughts can manifest in a variety of ways, but what makes them scary is that they are intrusive and unwanted, and they do not respond to one's efforts to dismiss them. For our purposes, the term "scary thoughts" refers to any worry, rumination, thought, obsession, misinterpretation, image, or impulse that feels inconsistent with whom a woman believes herself to be and causes a significant degree of anxiety or distress. It is an understatement to say that scary thoughts do not mix well with motherhood. The energy it takes to reconcile such conflicting thoughts at a time when women are exhausted and emotionally vulnerable is beyond description. Mothers with scary thoughts know only too well that it doesn't matter what we call them; they just want them to go away.

We are confident that a greater understanding of the nature of these thoughts will lead to better coping skills, less anxiety, and greater empowerment. The following classifications will help define the different types of distressed thinking, but remember that they are not mutually exclusive categories. Though the categories may have clinical significance when they are problematic or require professional treatment, most of the time these categories are fluid and overlapping. In other words, you might identify with one or more of the descriptions of distressed thinking patterns, shifting back and forth, depending on the circumstances.

You will find that our discussion of these categories will be viewed both within the context of postpartum anxiety and depression and outside this context because scary thoughts are known to materialize in either circumstance. In fact, scary thoughts are common for *all* new mothers and fathers. Also note that throughout the book, we refer to the term *postpartum distress* as one that encompasses symptoms of both depression and anxiety. It is our belief that the umbrella term "postpartum depression" does not adequately address the acute anxiety symptoms that often coexist. To be clear, postpartum anxiety can manifest singularly, as separate from depression, or together with postpartum depression. In fact, postpartum depression often presents as an extremely agitated depression relative to other depressive episodes, with anxiety as a predominant feature.

This is why women are often surprised at how anxious they feel if they've been diagnosed with depression. Some women believe that their anxiety is the most urgent symptom and don't feel depressed at all. Other women believe that their symptoms of depression are the most worrisome. Both states are characterized by high levels of emotional anguish, and both can present with scary thoughts. Regardless of the degree to which anxiety and depression manifest, we refer to them together as postpartum distress.

Excessive Worry

Many women joke that if they weren't worriers before they had their baby, they certainly are now! One new mother of a 3-month-old told Karen that there must have been something that passed through the umbilical cord from the baby back to her that she called "worry juice" that now ran through her previously calm nervous system. She said it felt as if a switch went off and that suddenly she began worrying about things to which she thought she would be immune.

Worry is a common process of contemplating situations that are believed to be dangerous and will occur in the future. When people worry, they are not only reacting to stress but also often catastrophizing about things that have not yet happened. As people worry about something that is either real or perceived, the arousal response tends to linger and can potentially impact other areas of their life.

Amanda said she was never a worrier until she had a baby:

> I used to be such a "go with the flow" kind of person. Nothing ever bothered me. But since Aiden was born, it's like my nerve endings are all frayed. Everything inside my body pulsates. I'm watching, I'm listening, I'm looking at things I've never seen, I'm hearing noises in the night that are coming

from nowhere, I'm walking into walls and falling over my own feet. The baby cries, and I jump to attention like a soldier ready for battle. What if something's wrong? What if he's sick? What if he needs to go to the hospital? It feels like I will never sleep through the night again. Sometimes all of this feels like God's greatest gift. Other times it feels like I'm imprisoned by my own life.

Everybody worries. Worry is a natural part of life that tends to soar dramatically within the unpredictable context of motherhood. At The Postpartum Stress Center, Karen's staff often comments on the openness with which she reveals her own tendency to default to worry. Even with adult children and an empty nest, Karen reveals that hardly a day goes by when she isn't worried in some capacity about one or the other "child." Whether they are driving a distance on snow-covered highways or craving homemade chicken soup to soothe their 102° fever, she never escapes the temptation to worry.

Under the right circumstances, with few external disturbances and the absence of compromising factors, such as those in the postpartum period, women can indeed worry "well." In fact, new research highlights the notion that worry may actually help reduce some of the negative effects of depression and fear by keeping the brain busy and by helping people plan and focus more efficiently (Engels et al., 2010). But when women become mothers and are flooded by urgent demands from all sides, worrying well often becomes a thing of the past.

Worry comes in all shapes and sizes, ranging from that which feels acceptable to that which feels exceedingly challenging. The situation, an individual's tolerance level, and her sense of vulnerability or control will combine to determine the degree of distress she might experience. For example, if there were a news story about a child who ran across the street and was hit by a speeding car, a mother would understandably begin to worry about walking with her barely 2-year-old toddler outdoors, wondering "what if" the same thing happened to her child. Her response might be to grab tightly to the hand of her fidgety child, though the identical walk yesterday prompted no such reaction.

Most people are accustomed to their own style of worry and are alert to when they may be worrying too much in certain circumstances. Worry becomes problematic when it begins to seep into other areas of functioning or when it is no longer an appropriate response to an anxious situation.

If that same mother felt extreme nervousness each subsequent time she walked her toddler down a street and constantly expressed her worry both by her words and her behavior, she might restrict their experience and create an impediment to her child's normal social and emotional development. Typically, as time and distance from the original worry event (negative news story) passes, the worry response (*I'm so afraid something might happen if we walk too close to the road*) associated with it should decrease accordingly. When it doesn't, it can spiral further down along the continuum of anxiety.

When worry becomes chronic, it settles in as a constant heaviness, often expressed as tightness in the chest, rendering it hard to breath. It is perceived by the individual to be uncontrollable and is on her mind the majority of the time. In this book, we refer to this degree of worry as *excessive worry*. When worry becomes pervasive, it can make people sick. The concept of "toxic worry" differentiates worry that feels proportionate to the immediate stress from that which may be an inflated state of fretfulness: "Toxic worry is a disease of the imagination" (Hallowell, 1998, preface). This is not to imply that people are making it up. Rather, it reinforces the notion that although there is a time and purpose for justifiable worry, there is also much excessive worry that results from wandering and creative minds that can't let go.

Such is the plight of many postpartum women. Though some do succeed in worrying well much of the time by responding to appropriate cues with acceptable levels of concern, for many mothers, this is not the case. For some, worry speedily cascades into a stream of steady unease, making it difficult to discern what is appropriate and what is excessive worry. Wondering whether the baby had enough wet diapers during the day is a common worry. Wondering if she will develop an eating disorder when she is an adolescent because she had fewer ounces of milk today than she did yesterday is excessive. In some cases, when a woman is vulnerable, everyday thoughts can overlap with disproportionate worry, setting the groundwork for scary, unwanted thoughts to emerge.

Rumination

When circumstances fall short of expectation, some people, particularly women, may begin to ruminate about their circumstances, their emotional state, and what this means. *Rumination* refers to the process of going over something in one's mind, again and again and again. Women who ruminate often focus excessively on the causes, meaning, and consequences of their distress, at the expense of doing something positive or proactive to address their situation. This "vicious cycle" can prompt feelings of hopelessness and despair, as they see no way out of their situation.

Consider the case of Lori, who began to ruminate over her moodiness soon after the birth of her baby boy.

> Everyone knows about postpartum depression, but this just seems so much worse. Why is this happening to me? I had an easy pregnancy; I gave birth to a perfectly healthy baby boy. Sure, I expected to cry a lot as my hormones got back to normal. But I can't even get out of bed. My in-laws have to stay at the house and do everything. I'm not giving my son what he needs. I'm a horrible mother. I'm such a loser. Maybe I should just disappear, leave them in the middle of the night because they will be better off without me.

Rumination is similar to worry in that it is a mental activity that can seem never ending. Both worriers and ruminators tend to interpret their life situations in a negative light and predict negative outcomes for the future. Like worry, rumination rarely leads to any definite conclusions about ways things can be better or decisions about how to approach life differently. In both cases, people end up feeling stressed out and ineffective.

The concept of rumination was initially used to characterize a thinking style associated with depression. Like Lori, people who ruminate are very hard on themselves and self-deprecating. Not surprisingly, this thinking style can lead to feelings of hopelessness and anguish. People who ruminate tend to reflect inwardly, focusing on themselves and their feelings of despair. Whereas people who worry (mistakenly) perceive that their worry actually helps prepare them for some looming tragedy, people who ruminate often believe that they are "stuck" and that there is nothing they can do to change their situation.

Recent research has shown that rumination is important in understanding anxiety as well as depression (Aldao, Nolen-Hoeksema, & Schweizer, 2010). In this book, rumination is conceptualized as another type of troubling thought that can be anxiety provoking for the mothers who experience it. In ruminating about the implications of their life circumstances and/or emotional well-being, some postpartum women, like Lori, draw conclusions such as, *My family would be better off without me* or *I'm going* to ruin my child because I'm a horrible mother.* These thoughts become particularly concerning when mothers become consumed with them, paralyzing them from taking actions that might help them emerge from the vicious cycle.

Obsessive Thoughts

Obsessive thoughts refer to thoughts, preoccupations, images, or impulses that are intrusive, persistent, recurrent, and difficult to control. Although they are almost always unwelcome, they are universal and experienced by most people. The invasive nature of these thoughts often gives them disturbing power, thus intensifying their impact and adding the *scary* component to a mother who is exhausted and doing her very best. Any new mother who is bone-tired, overwhelmed, and finds herself wondering if she is doing something the right way, for the right reason, at the right time, exactly the way others would do it themselves or expect of her, knows only too well how distressing these thoughts can be. Obsessive thoughts can be present as part of an anxious or depressive episode, or they can exist in the absence of any symptoms of emotional disturbance.

Anyone at any time can experience disturbing thoughts that seem to bombard them out of nowhere. This brings us to one of the most fundamental messages of this book: The factor that determines whether a thought is troublesome or not is not the content, but rather the individual's level of distress and meaning attached to the thought. One woman may think, *I wonder why the sky is so dark and ominous looking. Maybe there's going to be a thunderstorm. I better get inside with the baby.* Another woman looking at the sky might fear a tornado is approaching. She may then have haunting visions of her baby churning through the funnel cloud, swirling with debris up into the dark sky. She might then wonder whether having this thought has somehow increased the probability that it will actually come true. Here we see how the intrusiveness is not just due to the thought itself (the sky looks dark), but also due to the level of distress the thought evokes and the significance attached to it.

Elizabeth experienced frequent obsessive thoughts of harm coming to her newborn as well as to her 4-year-old. She stated:

> I can't ever fully fall asleep because I have these violent images that my baby has stopped breathing. What's more, this has now extended to my older

child as well. Recently, we went to the mall and parked on the top floor of the parking garage. My son started to run toward the edge, and I just had this image of him falling over the edge and splatting on the ground.

Because obsessions are so disturbing, mothers go to great length to get relief from them. Sometimes relief comes from avoiding the thoughts and images at all costs. More often, though, mothers find that they cannot avoid these thoughts and images, so they actively do something to neutralize them. Elizabeth, for example, checked her daughter at least 20 times each night to ensure that her chest was rising and falling. In addition, she rarely allowed her husband, her parents, or her in-laws to supervise either of her children for fear that they would not be vigilant enough to ward off a catastrophe.

As will be discussed at greater length in Chapter 3, these behaviors provide temporary relief because women feel reassured that nothing bad will happen. But, in the long run, these behaviors only serve to reinforce the strength of the obsessive thoughts because mothers do not learn that the catastrophic outcomes will not occur. When behaviors such as these are performed over and over to provide relief from the intrusive thoughts or obsessions, we call them *compulsions*.

Intrusive Memories

Childbirth can be a *physically* traumatic event because, in many cases, excruciating pain is involved. There can also be *emotional* trauma when women fear for the health and safety of themselves and their babies. Scary thoughts can present themselves in a minority of new mothers who experience a traumatic childbirth, and in these cases they take the form of intrusive and unwanted memories of the stressful events that they had experienced. Consider Angie's birth experience:

When I got to the hospital, they whisked me into a room but then left me there for what seemed like hours. I tried to ask what was happening, but the nurse and the resident said they couldn't tell me anything until the attending doctor was able to examine me. I was already experiencing a lot of pain. No one seemed very nice … Then, as I was delivering my baby, they saw that the cord was wrapped around his neck. All of a sudden, there was a flurry of activity; they were calling in all sorts of extra medical staff. I screamed, "Is my baby going to be all right?" No one would answer; it was as if they just wanted me to shut up. When I heard the doctor say, "He's not breathing," I froze. I thought I was going to lose my baby. It turned out that he was okay, but I can't get that sentence out of my mind. "He's not breathing, he's not breathing." And the whole atmosphere was so cold and impersonal—I can't shake that awful feeling.

Angie is struggling with *posttraumatic stress symptoms* associated with childbirth. Posttraumatic stress symptoms are prompted by an event in which there is a threat of death or injury of the individual herself or of a close other. Women who associate trauma with childbirth report intense fear, helplessness, pain, and a sense that they may lose control (Zaers, Waschke, & Ehlet, 2008). Mothers can experience posttraumatic stress symptoms in instances in which their health is threatened by labor and delivery but, more often, they occur when the health of their baby is threatened, and they truly believe that their baby is going to die. For women with a previous history of sexual abuse, the pain, feelings of helplessness, and perceptions of loss of control associated with childbirth can remind them of the abuse and cause them to reexperience the initial trauma.

There are three clusters of posttraumatic stress symptoms; these will be explained briefly in Chapter 4. For the purpose of this book, however, we focus on symptoms associated with reexperiencing of the traumatic event. Some people who endure a traumatic event reexperience the event over and over in their minds. The most common way in which traumas are reexperienced is in the form of intrusive memories. Some women who went through traumatic deliveries think over and over about the most distressing aspects of that experience. In some cases, women who experience these intrusive memories avoid caring for their infant because contact with their baby intensifies these thoughts.

Catastrophic Misinterpretations of Bodily Sensations

A final category of scary thoughts involves *catastrophic misinterpretations*—most frequently involving a response to bodily sensations. Some people have the tendency to notice subtle changes in their bodies, such as an increase in heart rate or a change in their breathing pattern. These people tend to be hyperalert to these changes and might interpret them as being dangerous or threatening. Undeniably, there are considerable physical changes that accompany pregnancy and the postpartum period.

Sometimes it is difficult to know whether an uncomfortable bodily sensation is a normal part of pregnancy and postpartum adjustment, or whether it is a signal that something is wrong. If it is interpreted as a signal that something is wrong, then it is typically accompanied by anxiety. When women repeatedly experience anxiety about physical sensations, they may avoid doing things because the anxiety is so aversive to them.

Stephanie began experiencing breathing problems in the third trimester of pregnancy:

> There were several times when I couldn't catch my breath, and I literally felt like I was gasping for air. I thought that there was something wrong with my lungs and, more importantly, that somehow I wasn't taking in enough air and that I would harm my baby. I was hysterical. The doctor explained to me that as my stomach expanded, it pressed against the diaphragm, but that it was normal and would not harm the baby. But still, I would freak out every time I had trouble breathing. Now that I'm 4 months postpartum, I still have trouble breathing from time to time, which is strange because I've lost a lot of weight. When that happens, I'm convinced that there is something horribly wrong with my lungs. That I'm going to die of lung cancer and that my baby will be raised without a mother.

Stephanie is describing thoughts that often accompany panic-like anxiety. She experienced a normal interruption of her breathing pattern during pregnancy, but quickly feared something terrible was wrong with her lungs, which proved to be an overreaction to the situation. In some instances, a person who has a powerful event like that is more likely to be on guard for similar bodily experiences and likely to interpret these in a catastrophic manner.

In these cases, physical and cognitive experiences may begin to interfere with a person's life; for instance, she may have frequent panic attacks and she may avoid going places for fear of having another. It's easy to see that if a woman is frightened about the way she is feeling and fears something terrible will happen to her while she simultaneously provides constant care for a newborn, the implications are multitude (*I won't be around to care for my child; what if something happens to me while I'm alone with the baby?*). Thus, catastrophic misinterpretations of physical symptoms can often prompt excessive worry about the woman's health and child rearing. It's hard for a woman to take care of a baby when she is self-absorbed with relentless and constant worry about her own well-being.

Stephanie describes the chain of anxious thinking that can drift between excessive worry and panic surrounding misinterpretations of bodily symptoms:

> I can't really tell if my worrying is a problem or not, but I can tell you this, I worry all the time. It's like I have this deep bottomless vessel of worry. If there's something to worry about, I'll worry about it. If there's not something to worry about, I'll make something up in order to fill the rest of the vessel. I know that sounds silly, but it's like if I find out something that I was worried about is now okay, I'll find something else to worry about. After I had the baby, I had deep cramping for a long time that wouldn't go away. I fixated on the idea that I must have ovarian cancer and if we didn't find it, I would surely die. I insisted my doctor order an ultrasound for me. While waiting to hear the results, I convinced myself that I had cancer and what terrible timing this was. How could I have a baby and now cancer? Oh my God! My baby would never know me. All I could think about was this pain I was having and how it was a new, unknown pain to me, so I was terrified. Now I have cancer? Is this what cancer feels like? I can't believe I have cancer now. That's all I could think. I could feel the blood rush throughout my body. Nothing felt right.
>
> Then my doctor called to tell me the results of my test were normal. I was ecstatic. For about 1 hour. I called everyone I knew and told them I was fine. Then, alone with my whirring head, I thought, so why then am I having this pain? If it's not ovarian cancer, what it is? It's colon cancer. And there I went …

In Stephanie's situation, we see how the domains of anxious thinking easily entwine. Here, excessive worry and catastrophic thinking interweave to create Stephanie's cycle of distress. Filling up a bottomless vessel with anxiety is a grueling endeavor. Sometimes it may feel as if the impulse to worry is as strong as the desire not to do so. Learning how to stop doing this is a skill that may not come naturally to some, but it can be achieved through hard work, practice, and dedication to the process and desired outcome.

FINDING PERSPECTIVE

Reconciling the manner in which a new mother can both adore her baby and torment herself with horrific thoughts has been an objective of researchers, clinicians, and mothers themselves, as well as the inspiration for poets and literature over the course of many years. It is beyond the scope of this book to explore the concept of maternal ambivalence or the social taboo of the darker side of motherhood. The heart of this book is to isolate the experience a mother has when she is stunned by the incongruity of her thoughts and her feelings and to help her better understand this disturbing phenomenon.

To help you with this process, Chapter 11 has been designed in workbook style so that you can integrate the information in this book with your own experience. You may choose to fill it in as you go; others may opt to leave it for the end. Your decision to read this and confront your fear is a courageous endeavor. You may be afraid if you do that, it will make things worse. It will not.

It has been described how the mind can "try to torment you with the thoughts of whatever it is you consider to be the most inappropriate or awful thing you could do" (Baer, 2001, p. 9). Lee Baer, PhD, Harvard professor and author, describes how a person's most vulnerable self can become engulfed by thoughts that cut to the core of his or her fears. To a mother, there is no fear that comes close to that of harm coming to her baby. This is an absolute. It is universal. It is primal. This is precisely why a mother is so susceptible and at great risk for scary thoughts. The unpredictable demands of motherhood, along with biological, hormonal, and psychological challenges, combine to generate anxiety and worry of unprecedented proportion.

Not all anxious thoughts are scary, and some women don't worry as much about this noise in their heads. They understand it to be part of feeling overwhelmed and are able to dismiss these thoughts without major difficulty. However, postpartum distress can manifest in copious fashion; it is frequently expressed as thoughts that mothers find unpleasant, offensive, or uncomfortable. Most people, at one time or another, have had a thought that scared them and wondered why in the world they would think such a thing. These thoughts or images or impulses may range from being mildly uncomfortable to vividly disturbing. This phenomenon appears to be part of the human condition. Fortunately, humans also have the capacity to compartmentalize these thoughts and protect themselves from these fleeting aberrations. But sometimes, for some people, under certain circumstances, the ability to filter these thoughts becomes compromised.

Motherhood is one of those circumstances.

Take-Home Point for Mothers. New motherhood is a time that is ripe for you to experience anxiety like you have never experienced before. Although it is normal to be anxious after the birth of your child, there are times when anxiety can be crippling. Anxiety following childbirth can take many forms—excessive worry, rumination, obsessive thoughts, intrusive memories, and catastrophic misinterpretation of your bodily sensations—and you will learn strategies for coping with all of these in this book.

Clinician Note. Although you have undoubtedly become more aware of postpartum depression over the past decade, only recently is attention being paid to the anxiety that a majority of postpartum women experience. Mothers can experience compelling anxiety, whether or not they are diagnosed with an anxiety disorder or depression. You can play a pivotal role in new mothers' lives by giving a name to the scary thoughts that they experience, normalizing this experience, and screening to determine whether your clients need professional help.

2

A Closer Look

If it's normal for new mothers to experience scary thoughts, how does a mother know what's okay and what's not okay? When should healthcare providers disregard scary thoughts as a typical response to the demands of new motherhood, and when should they treat them as a symptom of an anxiety disorder or depression? In view of the facts that postpartum moods fluctuate significantly and that a certain degree of emotional instability is expected, careful attention to the nature and impact of these scary thoughts is indicated.

Because postpartum women often spin in a cycle of worry over which thoughts are acceptable and which are problematic, you need to know if what you are feeling is a symptom of something more serious or if clarification and support would be enough to ease your mind. Ironically, one of the best measures is your own intuition. In fact, sensing that something might be wrong is a cue that you are in need of clarification. This does not mean that anything terrible is happening. Rather, it means that you are concerned about the way you are feeling and should follow up with your intuition to make sure everything is okay. Think about this: If your baby didn't seem "right" and you weren't sure whether you should take him to the doctor, but your gut kept telling you that something was a bit off, you would likely take him to the doctor just to make sure.

Likewise, if you don't like the way you are feeling or if you are wondering if something is wrong, it is time to do something about it. You may decide to try self-help techniques, nonprofessional interventions, or professional help. In any case, if you don't feel as if what you are doing is helpful, it is time to find someone who is knowledgeable and sensitive to the needs of postpartum women. In the absence of accurate information and true understanding, uncomfortable feelings and thoughts can swell into a deluge of despair. In this way, small bits of anxiety can escalate into persistent, scary thoughts.

Though the paradox of feeling simultaneously consumed by love and painful anxiety may seem inescapable, relief often can be found with self-awareness, information, and balance. It is worth restating that the specific thought you might be having, no matter how disturbing it is to you, is not necessarily the problem. The problem is how you interpret it, how it makes you feel, and how you react to the thought. This is why learning strategies for coping with scary thoughts is essential. We will see later in the book that wishing them away will not work, and feeling guilty about them only makes them more prominent. Learning to accept their presence disempowers them; ultimately, this becomes the greatest weapon in defeating them. So, with acceptance as the goal, we explore the nature, prevalence, common reactions to, and impact of scary thoughts.

THE NATURE OF SCARY THOUGHTS

The following points are presented to restate, reaffirm, and reassure. Given that the very essence of scary thoughts can be so disquieting by definition, we hope these points of clarification will provide perspective and much needed support. Identifying and putting words to some of the thoughts you are having can lessen the anxiety and ease the accompanying guilt.

- Scary thoughts are negative, repetitive, unwanted, and/or intrusive thoughts or images that can bombard you at any time. They can come out of nowhere.
- In addition to being a common symptom of postpartum anxiety disorder or postpartum depression, scary thoughts are a common phenomenon with all new parents (Abramowitz, Schwartz, & Moore, 2003).
- If you have a history of an anxiety disorder or depression, tend to be a worrier, or describe yourself as overly analytical or a perfectionist, you have an increased risk of experiencing scary thoughts. However, having no such history does not exempt you from experiencing postpartum scary thoughts.

- Scary thoughts can come in the form of ideas (*What if I burn the baby in the bathtub?*), images (*I keep picturing the baby falling off the changing table*), or impulses (*Every time I go into the kitchen, I feel like I'm going to pick up that knife and stab him*).
- Scary thoughts can be indirect or passive (*something might happen to the baby*), or they can imply intention (thoughts or images of throwing the baby against the wall).
- Scary thoughts are *not* an indication of psychosis. They may make you *feel* like you are going crazy, but you are not.
- Scary thoughts typically focus on your baby, but they can also center on you, your partner, and/or your other children.
- Scary thoughts can range from mild to unbearable.
- Scary thoughts can be intermittent or constant. They may be fleeting and manageable, or they may cause substantial life interference or distress.
- Scary thoughts can make you believe you are a bad mother. They can make you feel unfathomable amounts of guilt and shame.

Examples of Scary Thoughts

Keep in mind that these examples may or may not reflect the specifics of your own thoughts. Although it may be tempting for you to worry if the thoughts you are having seem worse or are not included in this discussion, remember that these are just a sample of what might be experienced. If the content of your specific thoughts feel scarier than those we have listed here, this does not mean you need to be more concerned. If reading some of these examples triggers too much anxiety for you, then skip over them for now. You might find, however, that seeing them in print confirms that others have also had these thoughts and that the thoughts have less significance than you have given them.

Thoughts can be about accidental harm:

- What if I drop the baby down the stairs?
- What if I leave the baby at the store?
- What if I drop the knife and cut the baby?
- What if the water is too hot, and I burn the baby in the bathtub?

Thoughts can be about your baby's well-being:

- What if he stops breathing in the middle of the night?
- If I take the baby out or let others touch her, she might get some disease.
- My baby is so fragile. There are so many germs and bacteria that could kill my baby.

Thoughts can be about intentional harm:

- What if I take this pillow and smother the baby?
- What if I press so hard on his soft spot that it crushes his skull?
- What if I take this knife and stab the baby?
- What if I get so mad I shake the baby?
- What if I throw the baby over the railing or down the stairs?
- What if I just drive my car off the bridge with the baby inside?
- I could just snap her little neck with such little effort.
- I could pull off his limbs and see the blood spurting all over the place.
- A chainsaw could slice his head right off.
- I could poke my baby's eye out.
- What would happen if I put the baby in the microwave or the freezer?

Thoughts can be sexual in nature:

- I'm afraid to look at his penis. What if I touch him and get pleasure from it?
- I might molest the baby.
- Every time I bathe the baby, I find myself staring at her naked body and wonder why I can't stop doing that.
- When I breastfeed my baby, sometimes I feel aroused. Does this mean I could abuse my baby?

Thoughts take the form of images:

- Envisioning your baby dead at the bottom of the tub
- Picturing your baby covered in blood
- Picturing your baby dead in the crib
- Imagining yourself tossing the baby out the window

- Seeing your baby lying in a coffin
- Watching your baby's funeral
- Seeing yourself smothering your baby

Thoughts can be about yourself:

- My children would be better off with another mother.
- I'm not sure I even love my baby.
- My husband would be better off without me.
- I can't live like this anymore.
- I don't want to be a mother.
- I don't think my baby likes me.
- I never should have had this baby.
- What if I feel like this forever and never get better?
- I'm not healthy enough to have a baby.
- What if the pain I'm feeling means I have an incurable disease?
- What if I never recover from childbirth?
- What if I die?

Thoughts can be about others:

- I don't trust anyone to be with my baby.
- What if someone hurts my baby?
- No one could possibly understand what I am feeling.
- Someone I love might die.
- Everyone thinks I'm a bad mother.
- If others knew what was in my head, they would think I am evil.

Thoughts can be about the future:

- What if things never get better?
- What if the baby does not gain enough weight?
- What if I can't handle going back to work?
- What if I choose a bad day care?
- What if my husband loses his job, and we lose the house and end up on the street?
- What if I'm a bad parent and ruin my child?
- What if my baby turns out to be a bad person?
- What if the baby inherits my anxiety?

Thoughts can be about the childbirth experience:

- I keep hearing them say, "He's not breathing."
- The nurse didn't care about me or the baby.
- The doctor didn't handle the baby very delicately.
- The pain was horrifying.
- I embarrassed myself by not being able to handle the pain.
- I thought I was going to die.
- I thought my baby was going to die.
- I can't bear to go back to that hospital.

This is not an easy list to read. As we stated earlier, the reason for including it here is to show that thoughts you might view as awful and horrific have also plagued numerous other women. Even though it feels like you are the only person who could dare to admit that you have had any of these thoughts, you are not alone. We know there is comfort for you in the knowledge that other women, who are similarly trying to be the best mothers they can be, are also suffering with these or comparable thoughts.

––––––

PREVALENCE

It may be surprising to hear that most healthy parents of new babies, both mothers and fathers, experience unwanted thoughts concerning their babies. Of the five categories we have been discussing, we have the most data about the prevalence of obsessive thoughts. Jon Abramowitz, a leading researcher who studies obsessive compulsive disorder, began to investigate obsessive thoughts in the postpartum period after he had his first child. According to one of his studies (Abramowitz, Khandker, Nelson, Deacon, & Rygwal, 2006), 91% of new mothers (and 88% of new fathers) experience obsessive thoughts about their baby at some point following their baby's birth! This means that almost every new mother experiences some degree of obsessive thinking. Most of these new parents experienced mild distress associated with these thoughts (Abramowitz, Schwartz, & Moore, 2003).

Research on the prevalence of intrusive memories of childbirth is accumulating rapidly and shows that approximately one third of women have stressful childbirth experiences (Creedy, Shochet, & Housfall, 2000) and that between 10 and 15% truly believed that they or their baby would die during childbirth (Lyons, 1998). One small study found that in 28 women who requested elective cesarean section, all of them had intrusive memories of a previous traumatic childbirth (Ryding, Wijma, & Wijma, 1997).

In a larger study of 592 women who had given birth 4–6 weeks earlier, 17% reported that they "almost always" experienced intrusive memories of childbirth, another 28% reported that they experienced intrusive memories of childbirth two to four times per week, and another 37% reported that they experienced intrusive memories of childbirth once a week (Creedy et al., 2000). A third study found that 14% of women experienced intrusive memories of their childbirth that were significant enough to cause life interference and distress (Czarnocka & Slade, 2000). Thus, intrusive memories of childbirth may not be as common as obsessive thoughts, but they affect a substantial minority of postpartum women and might be especially prevalent in women who went through a stressful obstetric intervention, such as an emergency cesarean section.

Less is known about the prevalence of women who experience excessive worry following childbirth. The key word here is *excessive* because *all* women experience some degree of worry as they adapt to parenthood. Amy's research shows that women who are approximately 8 weeks postpartum worry, on average, around 20–50% of the time about specific things like their own appearance, finances, the cleanliness of their surroundings, and completion of household duties (Wenzel, Haugen, Jackson, & Robinson, 2003).

To put this in perspective, people who report worrying about several different things at least 50% of the time often meet criteria for generalized anxiety disorder (described in Chapter 4), the basis of which is excessive worry. Thus, although we do not know the exact percentage of women whose worry would be considered excessive, we do know that the average postpartum woman worries about things at the level that is in the ballpark of some people who are diagnosed with generalized anxiety disorder.

If we have few data that speak to the prevalence of excessive worry in postpartum women, we have even *fewer* about rumination and catastrophic misinterpretations. Although we know that rumination is much more common in women in general than in men (Nolen-Hoesksema, Wisco, & Lyubomirsky, 2008), no research studies have examined the prevalence and course of rumination specifically in postpartum women. We expect that to change because, in our clinical experience, we see rumination as a significant factor that maintains postpartum distress in some new mothers.

Similarly, no research studies have examined the prevalence and course of catastrophic misinterpretations. However, we know that between 1 and 2% of postpartum women meet criteria for panic disorder (Wenzel, 2011), the anxiety disorder associated with catastrophic misinterpretations of bodily sensations that is also described in greater length in Chapter 4.

What does all of this mean?

- Approximately 4 million babies are born in the United States per year (Hamilton, Martin, & Ventura, 2009).
- If up to 91% of all mothers experience obsessive thoughts, this means as many as 3,640,000 women will experience this phenomenon!
- This figure represents only one category of scary thoughts: obsessive thinking. Although many of the 91% of women will also experience excessive worry, rumination, intrusive memories, and/or catastrophic misinterpretations, it is also likely that many of the remaining 9% of women who do not experience obsessive thoughts will indeed experience a different category of scary thoughts.
- In addition, the preceding figure represents only women who have live births and does not include pregnant women or women who have experienced pregnancy loss, both of whom are also at risk for scary thoughts.

In other words, chances are very, very high that a new mother will experience obsessive thoughts specifically, and chances are even higher that she will experience some form of scary thoughts.

Having a scary thought does not automatically mean that a woman has a postpartum anxiety disorder or postpartum depression. In fact, some researchers have found that the scary thoughts reported by women with postpartum depression were not any different from the scary thoughts reported by women who did not have postpartum depression (Hall & Wittkowski, 2006). What these figures do mean, however, is that childbearing women would be wise to be prepared for the possibility of experiencing scary thoughts and arm themselves with strategies for coping with them.

HOW CAN WE BE CERTAIN THAT SCARY THOUGHTS WILL NOT LEAD TO ACTION?

We have previously noted that despite the unsettling nature of scary thoughts, the actual content of these thoughts is less remarkable than the distress associated with them. Although a mother who is engulfed with the concern that her impulse to smother her baby with a pillow might take exception to this claim, it's true that the clinical significance is the *level of suffering*, rather than the content of thought itself. The level of suffering refers to the amount and frequency of the distress and how time consuming it is (Fairbrother & Woody, 2008).

As we would expect, if a mother perceives the thought as threatening, her anxiety is amplified. In this way, it is actually her appraisal—or misappraisal, to be precise—of the thought, rather than the thought itself, that ramps up the anxiety. She might falsely believe her thought is representative of her desire to make it happen—*If I'm thinking I could smother her, it means I want to hurt her.* Or, she might mistakenly believe that the mere act of thinking this thought might make it come true. That, as we've said, is a mother's greatest fear of all.

Unlikely Consequences

Could I actually do something to hurt my baby? A postpartum woman with scary thoughts worries constantly that something bad will happen. She worries that someone will take her baby away, and she worries that people will think she is a bad mother. But the dominant fear she holds deep in her heart is the fear that the thoughts are a warning that she will act on them and hurt her baby. This is not the case. In fact, research shows no correlation between a mother's scary thoughts and her acting on these thoughts (Barr & Beck, 2008).

Meg described her thoughts in her journal:

I don't feel like myself. My head is spinning with the most horrible thoughts. I'm sick to my stomach. Tell him to stop crying. I can't get these thoughts out of my head. I envision myself shaking him or grabbing him and throwing him down the stairs or out the window. The dark hours in the middle of the night are the worst. The world rests peacefully while I feel like I am losing my mind. I don't dare tell my husband; he will whisk my baby to his mother's house for sure. So he sleeps while I wrestle with my thoughts. Why did I have this baby in the first place? I am so tortured by this stubborn image of the perfect mother curled up in the corner rocking back and forth, unable to take care of her baby … is that me?? Oh my God, make these thoughts in my head go away.

I don't want to do this anymore. He won't stop crying. I won't stop crying. Thoughts are racing in my head with a vengeance. I keep spinning and spinning with stuff in my head, like knives and sharp things coming out of nowhere. I can't make it stop. Keep the baby away, keep the baby away.

Because of a postpartum woman's fear that she could take action or that these thoughts of harm to her baby might somehow come true, it doesn't take much to exacerbate her distress. Any reference, story, or news account of actual harm coming to a baby will resound in the mind of a woman who fears she and her baby might be next. They strike the vulnerable heart of a postpartum woman with scary thoughts because she often fears she will "snap" and do the unthinkable, something irreparable, something unforgivable. No matter how often clinicians may reassure an anxious mother that her scary thoughts are a normal phenomenon, the dread persists. Unfortunately, the media often reinforce this by sensationalizing the horror stories that pulsate in a new mother's mind, feeding her ever present worry.

Women who are concerned about the scary thoughts they are having do not hurt their babies. If you are reading this book for no other reason than to get that piece of information and validation, we will repeat this many times to make sure you don't miss the message. The anxiety that accompanies scary thoughts speaks volumes. Mothers who worry about the thoughts they are having, no matter how big and bad, are demonstrating anxiety that provides valuable diagnostic information.

It is understandable that you are frightened by these thoughts, but pay close attention to the explanation. When scary thoughts feel inconsistent with your belief in who you essentially are, your character, and your personality, they are referred to as *ego-dystonic* thoughts. When a thought is ego-dystonic, it is in conflict with whom you fundamentally believe yourself to be. This inconsistency creates piercing anxiety. However, this distress, as disturbing as it feels to you, provides reassurance that these thoughts are anxiety driven and not psychotic. In fact, your anxiety is an indication that you are aware of the difference between right and wrong.

We know that it can make you feel like you are going crazy, but you are not. Simply put, your worry about these thoughts is a very good sign.

Unfortunately, some healthcare practitioners may not completely understand this concept and may be equally agitated by the high degree of distress associated with the scary thoughts. This can inadvertently lead to rapid escalation of anxiety if the response is an overreaction or action that reinforces the mother's anxiety, such as fearing for the baby's safety. It is our hope that healthcare professionals make an effort to understand the unique nature of scary thoughts so that they can respond with appropriate compassion and level of concern.

Likely Consequences

If a postpartum woman who is concerned about her scary thoughts is not likely to hurt her baby, is there a cost to this high level of anxiety during such a critical time? The following sections examine the impact that scary thoughts can have on relationships and family functioning.

Avoidance

If we explore anthropological, sociological, or evolutionary constructs, we can trace generations of motherly love across many species that, without thinking, sacrifice their own food, shelter, or life on behalf of their offspring. Yet, in the face of scary thoughts, maternal instincts, as such, can become maladaptive. A postpartum woman with scary thoughts might fearfully respond by believing it would be best to avoid her baby. After all, she thinks, if she's having thoughts about harm coming to her baby, perhaps by staying away, she can keep her baby safe.

Meg was hesitant to trust her instincts and mistakenly believed that her baby would prefer cuddle time with someone other than herself. The avoidance of her infant generated a self-fulfilling prophecy. The more she avoided her baby, the more difficult it was to spend time with him, and the more necessary it became for another caregiver to ensure that her baby's needs were adequately met. Meg watched her baby responding to this substitute caregiver, who connected and formed a relationship with the infant. The attachment between the two that Meg observed served as "confirmation" of her distorted thought that her baby would be better off and happier with another mother.

This example illustrates the manner in which a woman's misinterpretation of a relatively normal experience can sharply twist out of shape, ultimately reinforcing her perception of helplessness. When this pattern persists, helplessness can spiral into depression. Scary thoughts do not always lead to depression, but, as we have seen here, lack of treatment and understanding can make scary thoughts a precipitating factor for a more serious emotional condition.

We have seen that scary thoughts, whether they manifest as worry, rumination, obsessive thoughts, intrusive memories, or catastrophic misinterpretations, range in degrees of duration, frequency, and intensity. When high levels of distress accompany these scary thoughts, mothers typically engage in avoidance behaviors or rituals in an effort to control their thoughts, to reduce the stress, and perhaps, above all, to make certain they will not act on their thoughts. It makes sense that women who feel out of control believe that staying away from the baby will (a) keep the baby safe and (b) reduce the trigger for their scary thoughts, thereby reducing their anxiety ever so slightly. What we see in its place is the undesirable reinforcement of the very anxiety they are trying to assuage. By avoiding the stimulus, they inadvertently empower the anxiety.

Mothers who use avoidance as a means of coping with stress are likely to be less responsive to their infants' cues than women who are able to confront some of their fears. Experts worry that avoidance can lead to infant stress and insecurities, potentially creating difficulties in parent–infant communication and longer term attachment issues (Murray & Cooper, 1996). (We discuss this in the following section.) Additionally, there is concern that avoidance behavior associated with a depressive response, such as irritability and disinterest in the baby, could impact the child's social and behavioral performance (Hipwell, Murray, Ducournau, & Stein, 2005).

Mothers who are tempted to avoid contact with their baby in an effort to reduce anxiety triggers should recognize that this will only make things harder in the long run. For Meg, the best approach was for her to try to spend small periods of time with the baby where she faced and tolerated her anxiety and learned that both she and her baby could benefit from that contact. Meg discovered that when she started out with small increments, she was able to increase the time with her baby gradually each day with less anxiety.

Attachment

As we've seen, highly anxious states can lead to behavioral interference, which can potentially influence the early relationship with one's baby. When women are reassured that their thoughts are within normal limits and actually not as scary as they feel they are, they believe they are better equipped to connect with the baby, despite their fear. Tolerating and pushing through the fear may be central to securing healthy attachments. In contrast, if a mother is depressed, she is likely to withdraw. If a mother is extremely anxious, she may be more likely to overprotect or overreact. In either of these instances, healthy attachment is an issue. Attention to the mother–child relationship is paramount when distress levels are very high.

Thus, it is believed that elevated maternal distress can have an adverse impact on the mother–child attachment. Maternal–child attachment refers to the emotional tie between the mother and baby, which is understood to have a direct impact on the child's social and emotional development. A secure attachment is formed when the mother responds warmly and consistently to her baby's physical and emotional needs. For instance, when she hears her baby cry, she attempts to soothe the baby. If the baby giggles, she may respond by smiling in return.

Although the research is inconclusive, some studies have suggested an association between significant distress in the postpartum period and the development of an anxious or insecure attachment (McMahon, Barnett, Kowalenko, & Tennant, 2006). Women worry tremendously about the possibility of an insecure attachment, intensifying their already anxious state. This leads to concern that their anxiety will "cause" them to bond insufficiently, destroy any hope of a healthy relationship, or—perhaps, the deepest injury—that their baby will not love them.

However, it is worth noting that distress during the postpartum period is not always associated with an insecure attachment, and oftentimes women diagnosed with postpartum distress are successful at providing optimal sensitive and loving environments. In fact, a study in which Amy was involved found that the relationship with the infant was one of the only life domains not to be affected by postpartum depression (O'Hara, Stuart, Gorman, & Wenzel, 2000). This suggests that women with postpartum depression go to great lengths to ensure that they are attentive to their infants' needs.

Sabrina, mother of two, said she had obsessive thoughts after the birth of her first daughter, but nothing compared to the incessant chatter in her head after her second daughter was born. She became fixated on the fact that each developmental stage the baby went through represented the very last time she would experience that precious moment. She refused to make plans with anyone that did not include the baby for fear she might miss something. At first, she was able to rationalize this because, after all, this would be her last child. But, as time progressed, Sabrina would get physically sick to the point of vomiting if she did have to leave the baby. Her husband thought this was excessive but attributed it to his wife's sensitive inclination and wasn't worried until she told him she wasn't able to shower without taking the baby into the bathroom with her so that she could keep her eyes on her.

In the cases of Meg and Sabrina, we see how irrational thoughts can set the stage for potentially unhealthy maternal–child attachments. Both women responded to their scary thoughts with behavioral extremes; one avoided her baby, whereas the other hovered. As unfounded as the thoughts may be, when a mother believes her scary thoughts, they hold the potential to disrupt her interactions with her baby.

Impact on Parenting

Understandably, women with postpartum anxiety and depression report higher levels of stress related to their parenting than nondepressed mothers do (Cornish et al., 2006). Imagine how this stress would be exacerbated for mothers who are also struggling with scary thoughts. Women who are suffering with guilt and shame related to the thoughts they are having are subject to huge misperceptions of their infants' behaviors.

For example, we've heard mothers tell us how hostile their babies are when the babies don't respond to moms' attempts to soothe them or how oppositional their toddlers are when they want to eat when mom is busy feeding the new baby. Very anxious mothers perceive their baby's behavior to be more disruptive or harder to tolerate than mothers who are less anxious. Or, an anxious mother may sense that her baby's natural response patterns are evidence that she is not a good mother. Research confirms that mothers with high levels of distress frequently perceive their babies as fussier than do mothers with lower levels of distress (Edhborg, Seimyr, Lundh, & Widstrom, 2000). It's easy to see how quickly responses can be misinterpreted when stress is high and thoughts become distorted.

Although it has been shown that high levels of stress related to parenting, coupled with low social support, can predict the presence of scary thoughts of intentional harm to the baby, there is sparse evidence of an association between these thoughts and harsh parenting conduct (Fairbrother & Woody, 2008). It makes sense, though, that women would be fearful about the potential link between thoughts of intentional harm and aggressive parenting (*If I'm having these horrible thoughts about my baby, I will be a horrible mother*). This has not proven to be the case. Even though scary thoughts can make a mother feel that she will do something horrible like abuse her child, we have found that women go to incredible lengths to protect their babies. Good mothers have scary thoughts. Good mothers with scary thoughts, who are concerned about these thoughts, do not hurt their babies.

Impact on Children

There is substantial evidence associating maternal distress with negative infant outcomes beyond those that have already been discussed so far. Even though this is disheartening information, it is nonetheless important to mention because this prospect can often motivate women to seek help if their distress is high. With specific regard to infants of mothers with postpartum depression, infants have been observed to be tenser, less happy, and more stressed than those infants of mothers without postpartum depression (Goodman, Broth, Hall, & Stowe, 2008).

Furthermore, there is a significant increase in behavioral, social, and emotional adjustment problems and some concern about decreased cognitive and intellectual functioning throughout childhood (Goodman et al., 2008; Murray, 1992). This association has not been demonstrated with regard to women with anxiety and scary thoughts, but it feels prudent to consider this potential impact. In light of these research findings, mothers should be encouraged to seek support if they are concerned about the thoughts they are having or the way they are feeling. When the distress is reduced, the risk of negative outcomes is reduced as well.

Impact on Marriage

Marital satisfaction is paramount at this time when both parents are at an increased risk for heightened levels of stress. The birth of a child will certainly amplify stress in any marriage, under any condition. The demand of steady, 24/7 infant care has a dramatic impact on couples and can provoke or intensify tension in the relationship. Adding scary thoughts to this picture can unsettle the relationship further. In an otherwise mutually warm and loving marriage, the presence of scary thoughts will introduce an unfamiliar and unnerving tension. This intrusion can sabotage even the most stable relationship.

Although it may seem too obvious to mention, many new mothers and fathers forget that any time one or both partners experience extraordinary distress, it will impinge on the marriage. What does this mean? It means the demands of a new baby and the additional stress of scary thoughts can affect the way the couple communicates, how supportive and respectful the relationship feels, and how well they problem solve and resolve conflict. Sometimes, couples are so busy tending to the needs of the baby that they unintentionally neglect the needs of the marriage.

Here, again, it is helpful to refer to research on women with postpartum depression, specifically, because the implications are pertinent to our discussion of scary thoughts. Women with postpartum depression report more marital tension, less supportive relationships, and poorer communication than nondepressed postpartum women do (Kung, 2000). It is not always clear whether this is a reflection of actual or perceived levels of greater tension, but, either way, it is significant. It has also been shown that the dysfunction in the marriage can persist long after the woman recovers from the depression (Roux, Anderson, & Roan, 2002). If we generalize these findings and apply them to women who are experiencing high levels of distress with scary thoughts, we can see how important it is to pay close attention to the marriage during this time.

One common theme that is evident in our clinical practices centers on resentment of the new roles and perceived division of labor: *He gets to go to work and I have to do everything* or *His life has not changed at all; mine has been turned upside down!* This transition challenges the couple's expectations, willingness to compromise, and ability to accommodate to the changing roles. The presence of scary thoughts will exacerbate this division, with anxiety piercing the relationship. The reason this is important is that couples need to address these feelings of resentment, which, if resolved constructively, will reduce feelings of stress and anxiety.

FINDING BALANCE

Coping with the distress of a scary thought often requires a delicate balance. This means you must weigh how bad the thought feels with one's own inner resources and capacity to identify it for what it is. Learning to designate the thought for what it is (*This is a scary thought* or *I am not my thoughts* or *Nothing bad is happening*) can help compartmentalize the thought as an entity separate from the self. In this way, rather than surrender to the fear, your "observing self" takes command. Having a trusted contact person who can help with similar grounding statements—such as, *Everything will be okay* or *No, we do not need to worry about this*—is one way to validate the reality of the situation and thus diminish the anxiety.

One of the problems with scary thinking is that it feels so real and, often, it's hard to tell if your thoughts are legitimate worries or if they are anxiety driven. In the middle of an anxiety attack, it feels as if the preoccupation is reasonable (*This time it really is a heart attack!*); without external verification, the anxiety and distorted perceptions can quickly intensify. Checking in with a contact person for ongoing confirmation can provide much needed reality checks and short-term relief.

In addition to having a contact person for grounding purposes, when you can find the strength and determination to share the details of your scary thoughts with a healthcare professional you trust, this can be a gateway to healing. In harboring these thoughts you know only too well how important it is that your healthcare providers understand the sensitive nature of these thoughts, as well as the appropriate response and intervention. If not, you may fear you are wasting your time, at best, and exposing yourself to ill-fated scrutiny at worst.

Keep these things in mind:

- Good mothers have scary thoughts.
- Scary thoughts are much more common than you think and are experienced by nearly every single mother at some time or another.
- The thoughts you have do not reflect who you are or what kind of mother you are.
- You are not your thoughts.

- If you are worried about having scary thoughts, these thoughts will not lead to action.
- The more you try to suppress these thoughts, the bigger they can get.

We have noted and will continue to repeat that all mothers and fathers experience scary thoughts in their everyday lives. Mothers remain the subject of this book because they are particularly vulnerable due in part to their biological and hormonal upheaval as well as to the constant stress of caring for a newborn.

Mothers who worry about scary thoughts do not act on these thoughts. There is no evidence to support that women with anxiety-driven scary thoughts harm their babies. Postpartum women take extreme measures to protect their babies from harm—in tragic accounts, even at the expense of their own lives. The fear of harm coming to their babies, particularly by their own hands, feels unbearable. This agony emerges as a natural response to a state of unspeakable anxiety. This response, however painful to experience as well as to witness, is precisely what clinicians should expect from a mother struggling with such intense anxiety. The acute anxiety associated with these scary thoughts is a clinical marker that should be reassuring to both the clinician and the woman who is seeking support.

Take-Home Point for Mothers. If you are having scary thoughts, do not be surprised by the strong emotional reaction you are having. This is understandable. Be alert to this emotion, but do not let it interfere with getting the clarification and support you need. Remember that no matter how scared you are, these thoughts are extremely common, and you can get relief by intervening on your own behalf and seeking help.

Clinician Note. Be careful not to overreact to a postpartum woman telling you she is afraid of her thoughts, particularly if she reveals thoughts that are frightening to both of you. The content of the thoughts is not relevant. Her level of distress should be a barometer with which you ascertain the seriousness of the situation. Immediate intervention includes solid reassurance and outpatient treatment or an appropriate referral.

3

Why Am I Having Scary Thoughts?

When a mother experiences scary thoughts, one of the first things she asks is, "Why is this happening to me?!" We've discussed that scary thoughts are present in the *majority* of postpartum mothers. Thus, one answer to this question is that scary thoughts occur because it is normal for mothers to experience them as they adjust to caring for a new baby (or another new baby). Although this may sound woefully unsatisfactory, it is nonetheless very true. It is happening because it happens all the time, to most mothers.

However, research shows that certain factors make some women particularly vulnerable to experiencing scary thoughts. None of the factors guarantees that a mother will have scary thoughts after the birth of her child. Some women have many vulnerability factors but do not experience scary thoughts, whereas others have absolutely no vulnerability factors, but are nevertheless tormented by scary thoughts. We view these vulnerability factors as increasing the *likelihood* that a woman will experience scary thoughts, as well as increasing the degree to which scary thoughts will persist and be distressing.

Notice that we have not used the word "cause." There is no research that shows definitively that any of the following factors cause scary thoughts to occur. Many women ask questions such as: *Did a chemical imbalance cause this? Or is it just me?* There is no simple answer to this question. We know from animal research that biology can certainly affect behavior, but we also know that behavioral responses that stem from certain environmental conditions can affect biology. Mothers who experience persistent scary thoughts might very well have elevated or depleted levels of certain chemicals, called *neurotransmitters,* in their brains, but it is impossible to know whether the cause is a preexisting "chemical imbalance," the scary thoughts themselves, or the stressful postpartum adjustment period. However, one thing is clear: Scary thoughts do not occur because a woman is weak or defective in any way.

Scary thoughts emerge from a complex system that involves genetics, biology, thinking styles, and environmental stressors. In any one woman, some of these factors might be more influential than others. To make matters more complicated, all of these factors affect one another. For example, biology, thinking styles, and environmental stressors cannot alter a person's genetics because genetics were determined at conception. However, the degree to which a genetic vulnerability is noticed in a person's everyday life *can* be affected by biology, thinking styles, and environmental stressors.

Furthermore, environmental stressors, like having to feed a newborn every 2 hours, can affect a woman's thinking. She might think: *I can't do this. I shouldn't have become a mother.* Conversely, thinking styles have the potential to make environmental stressors easier or more difficult to tolerate. The woman in the preceding example might be so distressed that she has trouble falling back to sleep after a middle-of-the-night feeding. But a woman who has the thought, *this won't last forever,* might feel less distressed, which in turn has the potential to be associated with fewer adverse behavioral reactions, such as sleep disturbance.

In this chapter, we describe the manner in which four main classes of factors—genetics, biology, thinking styles, and environmental stressors—make a woman vulnerable to experiencing scary thoughts. If this chapter feels too difficult to read right now, read only the parts that resonate with your situation. The following sections are filled with theories and research that may or may not be relevant to how you are currently feeling. Skim the chapter and read that which relates to how you are feeling. The important take-home point is that a number of factors may make women vulnerable to experiencing scary thoughts; however, as noted in subsequent sections of the book, a woman can take certain steps to increase the likelihood that scary thoughts are kept at bay.

GENETICS

No research has examined the genetic contribution to scary thoughts following childbirth—or scary thoughts that occur at any other time in a person's life, for that matter. However, much research has determined that genetics play a role in anxiety or mood disorders, which might or might not be diagnosed when a woman reports recurrent and persistent scary thoughts that cause life interference and/or substantial distress. Roughly speaking, the likelihood of inheriting psychiatric disorders like major depression, generalized anxiety disorder, and panic disorder is about 30–50% (Hettema, Neale, & Kendler, 2001; Levinson, 2006). Having a family member with one of the disorders makes a woman anywhere between four and six times more likely to have the disorder herself (Hettema et al., 2001). Even if a woman isn't diagnosed with a psychiatric disorder, having a family member with one of these disorders increases the likelihood that she might experience symptoms, such as scary thoughts.

On the surface, these statistics might sound daunting. However, there are important points of clarification to keep in mind. First, there is no evidence that a particular diagnosis is transmitted from family member to family member. Instead, what is inherited is the tendency to experience anxious or depressive symptoms in general, particularly in situations that are stressful. Second, having a family member who is diagnosed with an anxiety disorder or depression does not destine a woman to have one as well. A useful way to think about the genetics of anxiety and depression is to consider that each person inherits a range of emotional intensity and reactivity to stressful situations.

In Figure 3.1, we illustrate the genetic inheritance for anxiety and depression in three woman: Michaela, Jane, and Becky. We labeled the black horizontal line Average to represent the degree of anxious and depressive symptoms experienced by the average adult woman. Michaela has several family members who have been diagnosed with anxiety disorders and depression; thus, she inherited a range of emotional intensity and reactivity to stressful situations that gives her a higher than average likelihood that she will have problems with anxiety and depression.

Jane, in contrast, has only one family member who has been diagnosed with an anxiety disorder—a grandmother. The range of emotional responding that she inherited falls squarely within the realm of what would be considered an average level of emotional intensity and reactivity to stressful situations. Becky was born into a particularly resilient family in which no family members have been diagnosed with an anxiety disorder or depression. The range of emotional intensity and reactivity to stressful situations that she inherited gives her a lower than average likelihood that she will have problems with anxiety and depression.

There are two significant points of interest in Figure 3.1. First, because each of these women has inherited a range of emotional intensity and reactivity to stressful situations, her genetic history has determined a broad set point for emotional experiences like anxiety and depression. But there is a great deal of wiggle room within that range. Genetics do not determine one precise level of anxiety, depression, or scary thoughts.

Second, despite the fact that each woman has a very different family history, each woman's range overlaps with Average. Michaela, for example, might need to work harder to ensure that her mood remains near the average level than Becky does, but it does not mean that Michaela is doomed to struggle with anxiety and depression during stressful times in her life. In fact, the ranges of all three of these women overlap with one another to some degree, which means that they might very well appear indistinguishable from one another.

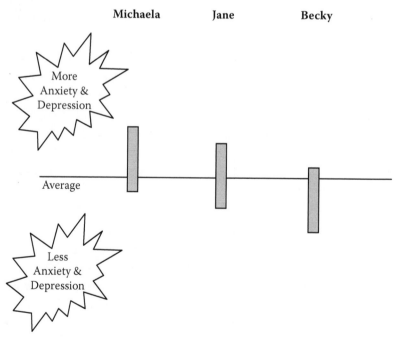

FIGURE 3.1
Genetic vulnerability for anxiety and depression.

We emphasize again that the research on genetics is mainly focused on vulnerability to symptoms of psychiatric disorders, rather than the occurrence of specific psychological phenomena like scary thoughts. This means that the degree to which the genetic research applies to the occurrence of scary thoughts is unclear, and we have to speculate on the basis of the available studies conducted to date on the genetics of anxiety and depression. All things being equal, scary thoughts are more likely in women who have a genetic vulnerability to anxiety or depression, and scary thoughts are more frequent and cause more life interference and distress in women who are struggling with these emotional disturbances.

However, as we hope we have made clear thus far, many women experience scary thoughts even in the absence of postpartum anxiety or depression or a genetic vulnerability to these emotional experiences. Thus, we view genetic vulnerability as one component that contributes to the understanding of scary thoughts reported by postpartum women, but it certainly does not paint the entire picture.

If you are a mother who is experiencing intrusive memories of childbirth experience, which might be associated with posttraumatic stress, you might be asking yourself how genetics plays a role in the development of your thoughts. After all, childbirth is something that you experience, not something that can be inherited. However, research shows that there is a genetic component to posttraumatic stress symptoms (Amstadter, Nugent, & Koenen, 2009), and intrusive memories are common symptoms associated with posttraumatic stress. This means that if a family member has been exposed to a traumatic event and subsequently developed posttraumatic stress symptoms, then you are at an increased likelihood of developing posttraumatic stress symptoms following an event that you experience as traumatic. There is no posttraumatic stress gene that is passed through generations. It is likely that what is inherited is the tendency for your alarm (fight-or-flight system) to be activated more quickly than it is for others without this genetic vulnerability (Amstadter et al., 2009).

BIOLOGY

It is well known that certain hormones skyrocket during pregnancy and childbirth and then plummet following delivery. Two of these hormones are *estrogen* and *progesterone*. Estrogen increases uterine blood flow, facilitates the development of milk ducts in the breasts, and stimulates the production of prolactin, which is a hormone responsible for lactation in new mothers. It also regulates levels of progesterone. Progesterone creates a viable environment for the baby to grow in utero, and it facilitates the cervix in creating a mucus plug so that bacteria do not enter the uterus. During pregnancy, progesterone keeps the uterus from contracting; at the end of pregnancy, progesterone levels decrease, which often corresponds with the beginning of contractions.

When levels of these two hormones drop suddenly, there is a potential for a corresponding decrease in serotonin (Beck & Driscoll, 2006). *Serotonin* is a neurotransmitter that is related to anxiety and depression, and scary thoughts are symptoms associated with both of these emotional disturbances. In order for messages to be transmitted in the brain, chemicals like serotonin must be transferred from one cell, called a *neuron,* to another at specific receptor sites. When there is not enough serotonin or the receptor sites are damaged, serotonin transmission is limited, and the likelihood of anxiety and depression increases. Thus, sharp drops in estrogen and progesterone are not directly related to scary thoughts, but they may make a woman vulnerable to experience cognitive and subsequent emotional disturbances by affecting serotonin levels.

Another hormone that has the potential to be related to scary thoughts is *oxytocin,* which is elevated near the end of pregnancy and during the postpartum period. Oxytocin stimulates smooth-muscle contraction during labor and plays a role in milk let-down during lactation. Most importantly for scary thoughts, there is evidence that oxytocin facilitates maternal behavior such as attachment to and nourishment of the newborn. It is possible that elevated levels of oxytocin overstimulate normal maternal instincts to protect the baby and keep her safe (Beck & Driscoll, 2006); one by-product of this would be thoughts about harm coming to the baby.

Much of the research conducted to examine levels of these hormones and postpartum adjustment focuses on depression, rather than on anxiety or scary thoughts. Moreover, this research has yielded decidedly mixed results: Some studies find that high levels of one or more hormones are associated with postpartum distress, whereas others do not. So, the jury is still out on the precise manner in which hormones affect postpartum emotional experiences. One researcher has speculated that postpartum distress may not necessarily be related to abnormally high levels of hormones, but that women who have these experiences are particularly sensitive to the major shifts in hormonal levels experienced during this period (Altemus, 2001). Just as with allergies, two women might go outside and one starts sneezing in response to the high pollen content, whereas the other has no such reaction. There may be similar disparities in hormonal responsiveness.

What all of this means is that the rapid rise and fall of hormone levels surrounding childbirth can throw you off balance physically, emotionally, and cognitively. Your body has already been taxed by pregnancy and childbirth, which compromise your psychological immune system. Couple this with the fact that some pregnancy hormones, like estrogen and progesterone, affect neurotransmitters associated with mood, and it is no wonder women experience emotions and thoughts unlike those they have ever experienced before. Women reading this book can take heart that the effects of hormonal shifts do not last forever; Amy's research shows that the prevalence of anxiety symptoms and disorders decreases across the first postpartum year (Wenzel, Haugen, Jackson, & Brendle, 2005), which also corresponds to the time in which most of these hormones fall back to their normal range.

Before we close this section, we'd like to include a word on premenstrual syndrome (PMS), which has been the subject of much research. Though the findings are inconclusive, it is clear that there is an association between premenstrual syndrome and the occurrence of postpartum mood and anxiety disorders (Garcia-Esteve et al., 2008). Research indicates that women who are vulnerable to premenstrual mood changes do not have abnormal levels of hormones; rather, they have a particular sensitivity to normal cyclical hormonal changes (Soares & Zitek, 2008) similar to the hormonal sensitivity example we referred to earlier (Altemus, 2001) regarding women who experience postpartum anxiety and depression. This means that PMS may be another biological vulnerability factor for anxiety, depression, and scary thoughts in the postpartum period because it signals a tendency to be sensitive to shifts in reproductive hormones.

THINKING STYLES

Of all the vulnerability factors discussed, the most research has been done on various types of thinking styles and their specific association with scary thoughts. Certain thinking styles psychologically predispose a woman to scary thoughts. Moreover, once a mother experiences scary thoughts, certain factors keep them coming back with greater and greater intensity. Unlike in the preceding sections on genetic and biological vulnerability, research has shown that some specific thinking styles make people particularly vulnerable to experience a specific category of scary thoughts.

Excessive Worry

Many women report that they have been worriers throughout their entire lives. Nevertheless, some factors increase the likelihood that worry may be especially evident during stressful times in a person's life. Research has identified four types of thinking styles that make people vulnerable to experience excessive worry (Dugas, Gagnon, Ladouceur, & Freeston, 1998):

- **Intolerance of uncertainty.** People who develop excessive worry have difficulty dealing with situations that are uncertain or ambiguous. They *must* know the answer or the outcome. Unfortunately, pregnancy, childbirth, and parenting a newborn child are fraught with uncertainty, so it makes sense that the postpartum period would be a time that is ripe for the development of excessive worry in new mothers who have a history of intolerance of uncertainty.
- **Inaccurate beliefs about worry.** Many people who engage in excessive worry truly believe that worrying prevents bad things from happening or that it will make them better prepared to handle bad things when they do happen. Most worries are unrealistic, which means that the catastrophic outcome about which a woman worries usually does not occur. Unfortunately, this ingrains the cycle of worry even further because it is easy to attribute the absence of a negative outcome to worry. Recall the description of Amanda in Chapter 1. She jumped to attention each time she heard a noise, worrying that something might be wrong with the baby. She held the belief that her hyperalert state prevented a tragedy from occurring; because nothing happened to disconfirm the belief, she was resistant to suggestions from others that she seek help to manage her anxiety.
- **Poor problem orientation.** A poor problem orientation refers to a person's lack of confidence in her ability to solve problems, even in instances in which she has perfectly fine problem-solving skills. It is

not surprising, then, that people who engage in excessive worry constantly second guess themselves, spend a great deal of time acquiring information on the issue about which they are worrying (e.g., excessive time reading articles on WebMD), and seek a great deal of reassurance from others. Although new mothers with a poor problem orientation think that their behaviors are helping to address the problem, in reality, these behaviors may take the place of quality time with children or much-needed self-care.

- **Cognitive avoidance.** Excessive worry can help people to avoid uncomfortable images of potential catastrophes because they are focused on the verbal *what-if* process. Although the short-term consequence of cognitive avoidance is relief, the long-term consequence is detrimental because the mental images quickly recur with increased strength, thereby intensifying anxiety and scary thoughts.

Mothers who have one or more of these characteristics before getting pregnant are especially likely to develop scary thoughts in the form of excessive worry after they give birth. Excessive worry can be scary because uncertainty is perceived as threatening. Inaccurate beliefs about worry are rigid and often hold women hostage. A poor problem orientation leaves women feeling ineffective, and cognitive avoidance increases the frequency and intensity of distressing worries, rather than decreasing them. These four thinking styles might seem impossible to overcome. As stated previously, many postpartum women who engage in excessive worry tell us that they have been like this their entire lives. Fortunately, there are specific strategies to address these thinking styles, which we explore later in the book.

Rumination

Unlike the other categories of scary thoughts discussed in this section, little research has identified thinking styles that predispose women to ruminate in stressful situations. Instead, rumination is, itself, a thinking style that in turn predicts psychiatric symptoms (especially depression), negative thinking, poor problem solving, lack of motivation and initiative, and reductions in social support (Nolen-Hoeksema, Wisco, & Lyubomirsky, 2008). In other words, women who have a tendency to ruminate during times of stress are more likely to get caught in the cycle of negative thinking and the consequences described previously.

Some research suggests that one aspect of rumination—the inability to stop ruminating about a mental state—is associated with especially high levels of distress (Raes, Hermans, Williams, Bijttebier, & Eelen, 2008). We think this aspect of rumination is what makes things feel particularly scary for mothers (specifically, rumination over the facts that they cannot stop thinking about how badly they feel and that they cannot get enjoyment out of their new child). And, perhaps most scary, mothers who ruminate foresee their distress lasting forever.

Obsessive Thoughts

As with excessive worry, a number of thinking styles predispose women to experience obsessive thoughts during stressful times. Researchers who have developed theories of scary thoughts in the postpartum period (e.g., Abramowitz, Schwartz, Moore, & Luenzmann, 2003) suggest that these thoughts take on greater importance and are associated with greater distress when mothers interpret them as threatening (e.g., that they will act on these thoughts). As we've seen, some mothers with scary thoughts demonstrate what is called *probability bias*. This means that they believe that thinking about a scary thought increases the likelihood that it will occur. Some new mothers who have scary thoughts demonstrate a *morality bias,* such that they equate thinking bad things with actually engaging in bad behavior.

Because these thoughts are so scary, many new mothers go to great lengths to avoid them. Although avoidance may be associated with short-term relief, in the end it reinforces the scary thoughts and makes them come back more frequently and with greater intensity. Many mothers hide the fact that they experience scary thoughts, which prevents them from obtaining evidence that these thoughts in and of themselves are not harmful. The avoidance and secrecy feed into a vicious cycle in which the obsessive thoughts become more and more consuming.

Three specific thinking patterns are associated with scary thoughts in new mothers who have never before had intrusive thoughts (Abramowitz, Khandker, Nelson, Deacon, & Rygwall, 2006):

- **Overestimation of threat/inflated responsibility.** Some women tend to exaggerate the probability and cost of threat and believe that they are responsible for causing or preventing the scary thought from becoming real.
- **Excessive need to control intrusive thoughts.** Some women believe that they must control all negative thoughts that enter their minds.
- **Perfectionism and intolerance of uncertainty.** Some women have difficulty accepting imperfection and have a need to guarantee safety or other positive outcomes.

Research shows that women who can relate to one or more of these categories of beliefs during pregnancy, when they are not experiencing scary thoughts, have an increased likelihood of experiencing scary thoughts following the birth of their children (Abramowitz et al., 2006). These same beliefs also increase the likelihood that women will have a negative reaction when they experience a scary thought (Abramowitz, Nelson, Rygwall, & Khandker, 2007). Because we know that most women experience scary thoughts after childbirth, it is especially important for women prone to these three thinking styles to be proactive in keeping them in perspective.

Intrusive Memories

Intrusive memories of childbirth usually present only in women who had a difficult childbirth, such as one in which they experienced much more pain than they had expected, feared that they or their baby might die in the process, or did not receive adequate care or support from medical staff. Nevertheless, research shows that some thinking styles increase the likelihood that women will have a traumatic stress reaction to childbirth and experience intrusive memories of childbirth in the postpartum period.

For example, research suggests that women who have a history of difficulty coping with adversity or who lack confidence in their ability to cope with adversity, especially labor and delivery, are at an increased likelihood of developing intrusive memories of childbirth during the postpartum period (Allen, 1998; Czarnocka & Slade, 2000). One of Amy's research studies demonstrated that women who believed that they would be able to use pain management strategies successfully during labor reported less pain during the early and intermediate stages of labor than women who did not believe that they would be able to use these skills (Larsen, O'Hara, Brewer, & Wenzel, 2001). Collectively, these findings suggest that perception of their inability to cope with adversity, discomfort, and stress makes women vulnerable to experience intrusive memories of childbirth during the postpartum period.

In addition, research suggests that women who are high in anxiety sensitivity are at an increased likelihood to develop intrusive thoughts of childbirth (Fairbrother & Woody, 2007; Keogh, Ayers, & Francis, 2002). *Anxiety sensitivity* is defined as the "tendency to respond fearfully to anxiety symptoms ... based on beliefs that these symptoms have undesirable consequences" (McNally, 1989, p. 193). Most women experience some degree of anxiety during labor and delivery, which is absolutely normal given the uncertainty and pain that they experience. However, it is possible that women who are high in anxiety sensitivity react especially adversely during labor and delivery. This, in turn, contributes to the perception of a negative birth experience, which then prompts the occurrence of intrusive thoughts about the negative birth experience.

Catastrophic Misinterpretations

Anxiety sensitivity is also relevant to understanding the origins of catastrophic misinterpretations of bodily sensations. When a woman who has high anxiety sensitivity experiences indicators of anxiety—especially those that are physiological in nature (e.g., rapid heartbeat)—the likelihood that she will make the catastrophic misinterpretation that these indicators are harmful increases (Austin & Richards, 2001). Thus, we view anxiety sensitivity as a thinking style that makes people vulnerable to make catastrophic misinterpretations when they experience a scary physiological sensation (difficulty breathing), a scary emotion (fear), or a scary thought (*Something must be terribly wrong with me*).

STRESSORS

Throughout this chapter, we repeatedly point to the fact that scary thoughts are likely to be experienced by genetically, biologically, or cognitively vulnerable women within the context of life stress. Regardless of the area of vulnerability, scary thoughts are much more likely to be experienced during a stressful time in one's life than during a calm period in one's life. Life stress can be associated with either positive or negative events. The key feature is that some change occurs that requires an adjustment period.

The postpartum period is a time of major adjustment for women—physically, mentally, emotionally, and relationally. Even in the best of circumstances when a woman is in a loving, caring relationship, her baby sleeps through the night, and the extended family provides just enough support to be helpful but also provides enough space so as not to be intrusive, the transition to parenthood (or parenting multiple children) is stressful enough to put women at risk for experiencing emotional distress. Mothers know very well that there are many components of postpartum life stress, including a baby that demands nearly 100% of their attention, financial constraints, and, oftentimes, decisions about whether or when to go back to work. Even when circumstances are fairly optimal, stressors can and do accumulate.

In addition to major life events that can be associated with stress, we also know that daily hassles can accumulate and increase emotional distress. *Daily hassles* is a term used to describe everyday stressors that cause minor irritation or frustration, like being stuck in traffic. Pregnant and postpartum women experience a number of hassles, ranging from strangers giving their tummies unwelcome pats to not having any clothes that fit. In her unpublished research on anxiety and postpartum women, Amy found that the total number of life events and daily hassles experienced in the previous year, which included pregnancy as well as the first couple of months of the postpartum period, was associated with the number of intrusive thoughts experienced by these women.

Stressors have different effects on different women, depending on the other factors described in this chapter. It often takes a lot of stressors to prompt scary thoughts in women with no genetic, biological, or cognitive vulnerability. In contrast, it often takes far fewer stressors to prompt scary thoughts in women who are vulnerable in all three of these other areas. All postpartum women share the vulnerability that is biological in nature because their bodies are adjusting to the rapidly changing levels of hormones, which in turn are associated with chemicals that regulate mood.

A BIOPSYCHOSOCIAL MODEL OF SCARY THOUGHTS

In Figure 3.2, we bring together a comprehensive model of scary thoughts. This model is very similar to one that Amy has proposed in her book on perinatal anxiety disorders (Wenzel, 2011). The word *biopsychosocial* means that biological factors (i.e., genetics, hormones, neurotransmitters), psychological factors (i.e., thinking styles), and social factors (i.e., life stress) are involved in scary thoughts.

The three circles on the left-hand side of the model represent the three areas of vulnerability. Arrows go directly from each of the three vulnerability areas to scary thoughts because we know that women characterized by these vulnerability factors are at increased likelihood to experience scary thoughts regardless of the stress that they are under (Ross, Sellers, Gilbert Evans, & Romach, 2004). However, we believe that the most common expression of scary thoughts occurs when a mother's vulnerability

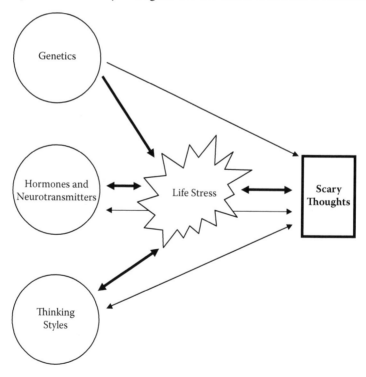

FIGURE 3.2
Biopsychosocial model of anxiety in childbearing women.

combines with the stress of the transition to parenthood. This is why the arrows among the vulnerabilities, life stress, and scary thoughts are represented by heavier lines.

Figure 3.3 integrates vulnerability factors for scary thoughts experienced by Michaela, the woman described earlier in the chapter who has several family members diagnosed with anxiety disorders and depression. In the "Genetics" circle, Michaela documented the fact that her mother has struggled with chronic depression for much of Michaela's life, as well as the fact that several family members have been diagnosed with various anxiety disorders. As stated previously, having several family members who have been diagnosed with anxiety disorders and/or depression increases one's vulnerability for scary thoughts in the postpartum period.

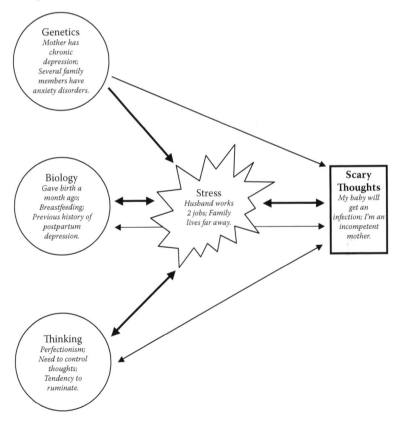

FIGURE 3.3
The origin of Michaela's scary thoughts.

In the "Biology" circle, Michaela recorded the fact that she is 1 month postpartum and is breastfeeding. She also noted that she had a previous history of postpartum depression, which increases the likelihood that she is susceptible to having emotional reactivity to the biological changes that mothers experience soon after childbirth.

In the "Thinking" circle, Michaela indicated three thinking styles that have the potential to exacerbate scary thoughts: (a) perfectionism, (b) a need to control thoughts, and (c) the tendency to ruminate. Michaela identified with these thinking styles even when she was feeling relatively good, but she also acknowledged that they became more ingrained in times of stress.

Unfortunately, Michaela was experiencing significant life stress at the time she completed this diagram, as evidenced by her responses in the "Stress" icon. Her husband worked two jobs and her family lived far away, making it quite stressful for her to care for two young children. As a result of the interplay among her genetic predisposition, biological changes, thinking styles, and life stress, Michaela experienced two prominent scary thoughts: excessive worry that her baby would get an infection because she was not thorough enough in caring for him and rumination over her belief that, as a result, she was an incompetent mother.

Figure 3.4 provides space for you to record the factors that you believe contribute to your scary thoughts. Do you have a biological relative who has had an anxiety disorder or depression? If so, you may have a genetic predisposition to scary thoughts. How long ago did you have your baby? The more recently you had your child, the more you might be experiencing dramatic changes in hormone levels to which your body might be particularly sensitive. Are you characterized by any of the thinking styles that could put you at risk for scary thoughts? What kind of life stress are you experiencing during the transition to parenthood? The stress could be specific to having a newborn (e.g., sleep deprivation, not even having enough time to take a shower!) or it could stem from other pressures in your life (e.g., financial problems, intrusive in-laws, your partner or husband having to go back to work). Finally, what types of scary thoughts are you having? Are they excessive worries? Rumination? Obsessive thoughts? Intrusive memories? Catastrophic misinterpretations? Write down your best guess in the "Scary Thoughts" box.

Even if you aren't able to identify any vulnerability factors or categorize your thoughts, remember that many women who have few, if any, vulnerability factors can experience scary thoughts. Ultimately, what matters most

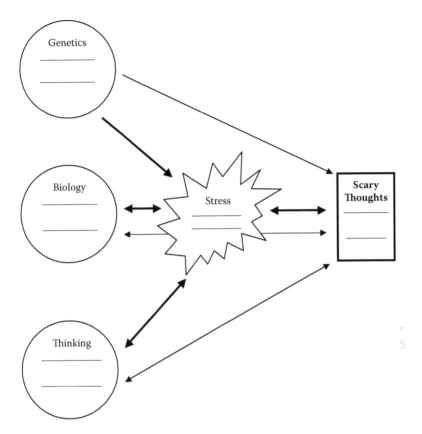

FIGURE 3.4
The origin of my own thoughts.

is that you recognize that you are having thoughts that are scaring you and that you are doing something about them. We know that these thoughts are disturbing, and what matters most is that you get some relief from them regardless of whether or not you can relate to the theories presented here.

Take-Home Point for Mothers. If you recognize some of these vulnerability factors in yourself, there is nothing inherently wrong with you. They are the logical expression of genetics, biology, thinking styles, and life stress. Although you can't alter your genetics, you can alter your biology (with medication) as well as your thinking styles and life stress. If you have been able to identify some areas that may predispose you to some of the anxious thoughts you are having, you are in a good position to determine the best course of action for relief.

Clinician Note. You may recognize the model that we put forth in this chapter: diathesis (or vulnerability) stress. Diathesis-stress models have been used to explain the etiology of a wide range of psychiatric disorders. Scary thoughts are no different. It can be helpful to consider a woman's personal and family history of psychiatric disturbance as you conceptualize her genetic vulnerability for scary thoughts. In addition, you might determine whether the woman has a history of mood disturbance associated with other aspects of her reproductive history, such as previous childbirths or menstruation. If your client experienced emotional reactivity in these circumstances, it is possible that she is especially sensitive to the fluctuations in reproductive hormones. Finally, we encourage you to be alert for the thinking styles that serve as vulnerability factors for scary thoughts. You can ask your clients directly if they are characterized by these thinking styles; however, in many cases, you can observe them in their interactions with you. If you determine that a client is characterized by several vulnerability factors, it will be helpful to educate her about the nature and prevalence of scary thoughts. Such recognition will go a long way in normalizing these thoughts and creating a comfortable and inviting environment in which your patient can share her experiences.

Section II

Clinical Concerns

4

How Do You Know If You Need Help?

At this point, you may be finding some comfort in reading the words in this book, yet you still wonder whether the thoughts you are having are really okay or if something is really wrong. Remember that, to a large extent, *you* are the ultimate judge as to whether the scary thoughts you are having are troublesome enough to warrant further attention. If you are not comfortable with the level of anxiety that you are experiencing along with your scary thoughts or if you are not comfortable with the manner in which scary thoughts are affecting your behavior, then it is reasonable to consider taking some action. Action could mean reading this book and implementing some of the coping strategies. Or action could mean seeking treatment from a mental health provider, such as a psychiatrist who prescribes medications or a therapist who provides psychotherapy. We discuss these options in greater detail in Chapter 9, so you will have some background information and guidelines in making an informed choice.

Many new mothers are so tired and overwhelmed that it's difficult for them to remember what is typical or they are not sure how motherhood is *supposed* to feel. These women would likely welcome additional guidance in evaluating whether they need to seek help. One way to determine whether help is needed is to consider whether your symptoms are frequent and/or intense enough to warrant a psychiatric diagnosis. This chapter describes symptoms of the psychiatric disorders that can, in some instances, underlie the expression of scary thoughts and that have been shown to benefit from professional help. Although the precise diagnosis may not be relevant here, it will be helpful for you to begin to understand how your thinking patterns might contribute to the larger clinical picture. Even in the absence of a diagnosis of one of the disorders described here, you may still be experiencing scary thoughts that are very distressing to you. This distress is often reason enough for you to seek help.

Understandably, you may be reluctant to accept the possibility of a psychiatric diagnosis. Bear in mind that these disorders will not describe everyone reading this book and are not intended to be used for self-diagnosis. They are clinical distinctions that may serve to guide you in your effort toward greater understanding and relief. Even if it appears that you have every single symptom associated with one or more of the psychiatric disorders described, it is best for a healthcare professional to verify the diagnosis. When making a psychiatric diagnosis, healthcare professionals not only consider the presence or absence of a symptom but also evaluate the intensity of the symptoms, the percentage of time the symptoms are experienced, and the degree to which the symptoms cause life interference or emotional distress.

The following sections describe five psychiatric disorders for which mothers may seek help, including:

- Generalized anxiety disorder
- Depression
- Obsessive compulsive disorder
- Posttraumatic stress disorder
- Panic disorder

The key with each of these disorders is that the more the symptoms cause life interference or emotional distress, the more we would encourage seeking help. Life interference might take the form of the consequences of scary thoughts we described in Chapter 2, such as avoidance or overprotection of your baby. As we've noted, emotional distress means that you are significantly bothered by having the symptoms.

Toward the end of the chapter, we review two types of scary thoughts for which we suggest that you seek help immediately: suicidal thoughts and psychotic thoughts. We are hopeful that this information will lead you toward a deeper understanding of your distress in order to help you find relief from your suffering. If, however, this chapter feels as if it's too much clinical information for you to absorb right now or if it feels irrelevant to your experience, we encourage you to skip over it and read only the parts of the book that feel pertinent and helpful to you.

GENERALIZED ANXIETY DISORDER

The key feature of generalized anxiety disorder (GAD) is excessive worry, which is one of the categories of scary thoughts that we introduced in Chapter 1. Women with GAD find that they spend more of their time worrying than not worrying. When they worry, they find that they have difficulty controlling it. They are inundated with endless streams of *what-if* questions. Their worries are big (*What if my child develops an incurable disease?*) and small (*What if I have trouble consoling my child while we are out in public today?*). Regardless of whether the worries are big or small, people with GAD estimate that the feared consequences will be intolerable and that they will not have the ability to cope with them.

Worry is a part of human nature; what distinguishes women with GAD is that the worry is pervasive, associated with life interference and/or emotional distress, and associated with a number of specific symptoms. These specific symptoms include restlessness, being easily fatigued, difficulty concentrating, irritability, muscle tension, and sleep disturbance (in the case of new mothers, sleep disturbance in excess of what typically occurs when a newborn wakes multiple times throughout the night). It is not necessary for all these symptoms to be present in order to be diagnosed with GAD. Typically, GAD diagnoses are assigned when someone reports the experience of excessive, uncontrollable worry, more of the time than not, that is accompanied by at least three of the aforementioned symptoms.

Although much of the excessive worry described in this book focuses on worry about the health and relationship with the new baby, in truth, postpartum women with GAD worry about all kinds of things. Some women worry about their relationships with their older child, believing that this child is not getting enough attention because they are consumed with their newborn. Other women worry about finances and whether they will be able to make ends meet now that the baby has arrived. Women who work worry about what their life will be like after their maternity leave is over, such as whether they will be able to handle their job, whether they will find their day care to be adequate, or whether they will be able to leave their babies. In most cases, the worries seem endless.

The life interference and emotional distress experienced by postpartum women with GAD can be considerable. Many women report frequent disagreements with their partners as they wonder how their partners can possibly be so calm in the midst of so many things that can go wrong. Some women are highly irritated that their partners are not assuming their fair share of the worry. Conflict with or negative feelings toward one's partner have the potential to create a situation in which the new mother feels unsupported, and the couple no longer functions as a team.

Symptoms of GAD can also interfere with getting things done. For example, fatigue and difficulty concentrating can make it difficult to meet work responsibilities, balance a checkbook, or plan a family gathering. Even if excessive worry and its associated symptoms do not get in the way of a mother's relationships, work performance, or ability to manage the household, they can nevertheless cause sizeable emotional distress. Many women with GAD report that they are unhappy and unable to appreciate the precious moments with their baby. Not surprisingly, many women with GAD also struggle with depression (Wenzel, 2011).

Consider Amanda, who was introduced in Chapter 1. Before having her child, she regarded herself as easygoing and laid back; now, she is constantly on edge. This is what she had to say about the associated symptoms and consequences of her excessive worry:

> It's to the point that I'm so tired, I'm just like a zombie. I try to lie down when Aiden takes a nap, but I usually can't sleep. It's almost the opposite— as soon as my attention is no longer focused on Aiden, my mind starts racing with all of the things I need to get done. It's ironic that I'm so concerned about my ever growing list, but I never actually get things done. My husband tries to be understanding, but he's at the end of his rope. He says he can't do much more after working over 8 hours a day, 5 days a week and having as much responsibility around the house that he does. I'm so afraid that this will never end, that I'm irreversibly scarred after having the baby.

Amanda sought treatment with a psychotherapist when she was 9 months postpartum; at that time, she was diagnosed with GAD.

One technical point about a diagnosis of GAD is in order here. According to the *Diagnostic and Statistical Manual of Mental Disorders* (4th ed., text revision; DSM-IV-TR; APA, 2000), a person is diagnosed with GAD only if she has reported excessive worry and associated symptoms for at least 6 months. Most people who are diagnosed with GAD have experienced excessive worry for a very long time and often describe themselves as lifelong worriers.

Amy's research suggests that two main groups of women are diagnosed with postpartum GAD (Wenzel, Haugen, Jackson, & Robinson, 2003). The first group is similar to the people described previously: They report that they have always been prone to worry but that their worry became much more excessive and uncontrollable during pregnancy and/or following childbirth. The second group experiences a sudden onset of excessive worry and associated symptoms, usually soon after the birth of their child. However, in many cases these women have not experienced this degree of worry for a full 6-month period. Women in the second group who choose to seek help for excessive worry may be diagnosed with an *adjustment disorder* rather than GAD. Regardless of the specific diagnosis, treatment will be the same. For example, if a woman seeks psychotherapy, her therapist will target the excessive worry and the emotional distress that it causes, in order to help her find relief.

DEPRESSION

Postpartum depression (PPD) is an umbrella term often used to describe the majority of mood disorders that can emerge during the postpartum period. For the purpose of our discussion, we focus on women who have symptoms of *major depressive disorder* and refer to this as postpartum depression, whereas our use of the phrase "postpartum distress" encompasses both depression and anxiety. Many symptoms contribute to a diagnosis of postpartum depression, including:

- Depressed mood
- Lack of engagement in pleasurable activities or the inability to experience pleasure
- Appetite disturbance (either eating too little or too much)
- Sleep disturbance (either sleeping too little or too much)
- Psychomotor agitation (e.g., fidgeting) or retardation (e.g., moving more slowly than normal)
- Fatigue
- Perception of worthlessness and/or inappropriate guilt
- Difficulty concentrating and/or indecisiveness
- Recurrent thoughts of death, suicidal thoughts, and/or suicidal behavior (e.g., a suicide attempt)

Postpartum depression is usually diagnosed when a woman struggles with at least five of these symptoms for at least a 2-week period and the symptoms cause life interference and/or emotional distress. Though at times it can be confusing to distinguish, symptoms of this intensity and duration are strikingly different from the "baby blues." The blues, which occur in up to 85% of all postpartum women, emerge within the first 2 or 3 weeks following childbirth (Nonacs, 2006). Characterized by mood instability (e.g., emotional lability, weepiness), the blues subside on their own and require no intervention other than reassurance and some extra rest. If symptoms last more than 2 or 3 weeks, women are at greater risk for more serious postpartum distress.

Because the normal changes during the postpartum period closely overlap with symptoms of depression, the diagnosis of postpartum depression is often difficult and, at times, easy to miss. For example, women with newborns get very little sleep and are constantly exhausted. Some mothers have difficulty concentrating on mundane details or find they cannot make what used to be a simple decision. Trained mental health professionals rely on standard questions to determine whether new mothers meet criteria for postpartum depression:

- Are the symptoms in excess of what is experienced by most new mothers?
- Are the symptoms considerably different from the woman's usual level of functioning?
- Do the symptoms persist even when they are less likely to be explained by the demands of new parenthood (e.g., whether she is able to sleep when her baby is sleeping)?

Postpartum depression can make an already stressful period of time seem almost impossible to navigate. Some women with postpartum depression view themselves as doing the bare minimum to care for their children and keep their households running. Although exhausted and depleted, postpartum women forge forward to care for their babies and others who may need them. As Karen notes:

Women who are severely ill can present well and look good. Really good. At first glance, they can look good physically with every hair in place, and they can look good clinically, responding to our questions with deliberate precision. Unremitting symptoms of depression might be lurking behind the camouflage that things are fine. If clinicians aren't carefully reading between the lines at all times, they might miss that. (Kleiman, 2008, p. 3)

We see how, to outside observers, a mother may appear to be functioning just fine, despite the fact that she is depleted and believes she has hit rock bottom.

The type of scary thought that we link most closely with depression is rumination because research shows that rumination is a feature of people with depression, particularly women (Nolen-Hoeksema, Wisco, & Lyubormirsky, 2008). Some research suggests that rumination can exacerbate the course of a major depressive episode (e.g., Nolen-Hoeksema, Morrow, & Frederickson, 1993), in part because it feeds into one's sense of worthlessness and excessive guilt.

Although rumination might possibly be the most common form of scary thoughts that are associated with postpartum depression, all of the scary thoughts described in this book are relevant. For example, some research shows that between 41 and 57% of women with postpartum depression reported aggressive thoughts of harming their babies (Jennings, Ross, Popper, & Elmore, 1999; Wisner, Peindl, Gigliotti, & Hanusa, 1999), which we regard as obsessive thoughts. As stated, symptoms of GAD and symptoms of major depressive disorder overlap a great deal, and research shows that postpartum women who report symptoms of depression also experience high levels of worry (Austin, Tully, & Parker, 2007). As noted earlier, most women with postpartum depression present in an agitated state characterized by both anxiety and depression.

Lori, whom we introduced in Chapter 1 when we described rumination, was experiencing postpartum depression. She reported symptoms of depressed mood, inability to experience pleasure, overeating, oversleeping, a perception of worthlessness, excessive guilt, and difficulty concentrating. This is how she described the impact of her depressive symptoms on her life and the manner in which they exacerbated her scary, ruminative thoughts:

I'm failing my son, and I'm failing my husband. I'm pathetic. My son is happier to be around my in-laws than he is to be around me. But I can't get up the energy to do anything about it. I'm supposed to be back to work, but there is no way I can focus long enough to sit at a computer. As a result, my husband and I are taking a big financial hit, which only makes me feel guiltier. I can't believe the patience that my husband and in-laws have with me. I don't deserve it. I can't get it out of my mind that I am a horrible person and that I deserve to suffer.

Lori's rumination (e.g., focusing on failing her family, labeling herself as pathetic and as a horrible person) probably only made her depression that much more difficult to bear and entrenched her in the cycle of negative thoughts and overwhelming emotions. Many women report that depression, anxiety, and scary thoughts develop several weeks or months following childbirth. When this happens, it sometimes corresponds to a stressful event associated with the transition to parenthood, such as going back to work, or a major loss, but not always. Though the current diagnostic standard for postpartum major depressive disorder requires onset within the first 4 weeks following childbirth (DSM-IV-TR; APA, 2000), most experts on this subject define the postpartum period as being much longer, oftentimes the entire first year following delivery (Beck & Driscoll, 2006; Kleiman & Raskin, 1994; Wenzel, 2011).

At the time of this writing, the proposed revision of the DSM (i.e., DSM-V) expands this 4-week specifier of postpartum onset from 4 weeks to 6 months. This is certainly a step in the right direction. Still, regardless of the time frame set forth by clinical guidelines, when you are feeling bad, it's bad, no matter what anyone labels it. There can also be a sense that you always have, and always will, feel this way. What is critical at this point in time is that you connect with a knowledgeable professional with whom you feel comfortable. Regardless of when your symptoms of depression emerged, the immediate goal is to find symptom relief and reduce the impact the depression is having on your life.

OBSESSIVE COMPULSIVE DISORDER

As indicated by its name, obsessive compulsive disorder (OCD) is characterized by two main features: obsessions and compulsions. *Obsessions* are the obsessive thoughts that were defined in Chapter 1, which are intrusive thoughts, images, or urges that are disturbing and inconsistent with whom a person believes herself to be. *Compulsions* are behaviors in which a person must engage repeatedly, in many instances to neutralize the obsessions. A woman is diagnosed with OCD when she presents with obsessions or compulsions and the symptoms cause life interference, emotional distress, and/or are time consuming (i.e., take more than an hour per day).

Despite its name, a person does not have to experience *both* obsessions and compulsions; in fact, many people who are diagnosed with OCD have only one or the other. This fact is especially relevant to new mothers because some researchers have suggested that postpartum women who are diagnosed with OCD primarily report obsessions (Sichel, Cohen, Rosenbaum, & Driscoll, 1993).

Obsessive compulsive symptoms can take many forms. Abramowitz, Schwartz, and Moore (2003) sorted the typical obsessive thoughts of postpartum women into seven categories:

- Thoughts of suffocation or SIDS
- Thoughts of accidents
- Ideas or urges of intentional harm
- Thoughts of losing the baby
- Illness
- Unacceptable sexual thoughts
- Contamination

The majority of obsessive thoughts experienced in the postpartum period pertain to the new baby.

Women who demonstrate compulsive behavior following childbirth usually fall into one of two categories: those who check excessively (usually to prevent a catastrophe, such as harm coming to the baby) or those who wash or clean excessively (usually to prevent contamination of the baby) (Uguz, Akman, Kaya, & Cilli, 2007). Two other categories of compulsions often seen in people who are diagnosed with OCD (counting and hoarding) are not generally observed in postpartum women. Typically, when counting and hoarding are observed in new mothers, the behaviors were already practiced before the baby was born.

Elizabeth, the new mother described in Chapter 1 who experienced violent images of her children's deaths, reported a high frequency of distressing obsessive thoughts, which led to the diagnosis of OCD. The life interference that is typical of a diagnosis of OCD can include things like elaborate rituals to check that the baby's furniture, accessories, and toys are safe or avoiding almost all contact with the baby to ensure that he comes to no harm. In other words, life interference is acknowledged when a new mother changes her behavior so markedly that it disrupts her or her family's usual functioning. Elizabeth's symptoms were associated with noticeable life interference because she was exhausted by checking on her newborn frequently during the night but would not allow anyone to help her watch the children during the day for fear that no one could monitor the children closely enough.

It may be helpful here to make the distinction between actual obsessions and excessive worry about real-life problems. In fact, it is often extremely difficult to differentiate between excessive worries and obsessions. Amy recently did an analysis of the similarities and differences between excessive worries and obsessions (Wenzel, 2011). Excessive worries are more likely to be realistic and pertain to everyday situations (*What if my baby does not sleep through the night?*), whereas obsessive thoughts are less likely to be realistic and more likely to pertain to events or situations that occur less often (*What if I stab my baby with a knife while I'm cooking?*).

The consequences of excessive worry are often less serious than the consequences of obsessive thoughts (e.g., getting a sleepless night vs. the death of one's child). In addition, some research suggests that people engage in chronic worry to avoid vivid images of feared outcomes (Borkovec & Inz, 1990); this fuels the cycle of worry because it prevents people from confronting their worst fears. In contrast, people with obsessive thoughts often report that their thoughts are associated with horrifying images.

Although these distinctions are useful for classification purposes, the boundary between excessive worries and obsessions is often blurred, and many scary thoughts fall into a gray area with characteristics of both excessive worries and obsessions. The bottom line is that it doesn't matter if you are having trouble classifying your thoughts as excessive worries or obsessions. Both are common, both are scary, and both can be managed using the strategies described in this book and through professional intervention.

POSTTRAUMATIC STRESS DISORDER

Posttraumatic stress disorder (PTSD) is an anxiety disorder that can occur when a person experiences or witnesses the actual or threatened death or serious injury of herself or another. When a woman endures such an event, she often reacts with significant fear, horror, or feelings of help-lessness. These two features—witnessing an event involving death and reacting with horror—contribute to the definition of whether a person has experienced a *trauma*.

Interestingly, whether or not childbirth constitutes a traumatic event has been the subject of some debate. In previous editions of the mental health professionals' diagnostic system, it was specified that a trauma was only a trauma if it was an event that was outside the range of the typical human experience (Bailham & Joseph, 2003). Childbirth would not have fallen in that category because the majority of women give birth at some point during their childbearing years. However, this viewpoint has changed, and it is now acknowledged that childbirth can be trau-matic for women and that some women develop PTSD as a result of this experience. Specific aspects of childbirth that are traumatic for women include emergency cesarean section, one's partner not being present for labor, a perception of not being in control of the pain, expectations that the baby will be harmed, and perceived lack of support from medical staff (Wenzel, 2011).

Clinically speaking, individuals must exhibit three "clusters" of symp-toms to be diagnosed with PTSD, and scary thoughts are one of the symp-toms in one of these categories. One cluster of symptoms pertains to the reexperiencing of the trauma. A diagnosis of PTSD requires that people experience intrusive memories of the trauma, nightmares or flashbacks about the trauma, and/or emotional or physical distress when something reminds them of the trauma. In this way, scary thoughts about a woman's childbirth experience are a form of reexperiencing it.

The second cluster of symptoms involves emotional numbing and avoidance of reminders of the trauma. At least three of these avoidance and numbing symptoms are required for a PTSD diagnosis, including efforts to avoid reminders of the trauma, difficulty remembering aspects of the trauma, diminished interest in pleasurable activities, detachment from others, a restricted range of emotions, and a sense that the future will somehow be cut short. Finally, the third cluster of symptoms per-tains to indicators of increased arousal or anxiety. Symptoms for PTSD in this cluster include increased arousal symptoms, such as sleep distur-bance, irritability or anger, concentration difficulties, hypervigilance (i.e., the tendency to be on guard and scan the environment for threat), and a heightened startle response.

Though intrusive memories of the trauma are a central feature of the clinical presentation of PTSD, plenty of women who have intrusive and unpleasant memories of childbirth do not meet full diagnostic criteria for the disorder. Even without the diagnosis of PTSD, these memories can be disturbing and are associated with increased anxiety (Czarnocka & Slade, 2000).

Again, if the symptoms you are experiencing are troubling you, it may be comforting to know that, with or without a diagnosis, you can get relief from these symptoms. It is worth reiterating that the level of stress or disturbance in functioning caused by symptoms is the best indicator of the need for evaluation.

Angie, the new mother described in Chapter 1, reexperienced her traumatic childbirth experience many times during the day, often finding that she was not able to maintain focus on a variety of tasks throughout the day. As she tried desperately to avoid reminders of childbirth, she reported feeling detached from her baby and sometimes resentful that her baby was the reason she was feeling so bad. In time, this detachment was accompanied by avoidance behaviors that kept Angie at a distance from her baby. She reported increased startle when something jarred her away from her intrusive memory, though she claimed to have no memory of certain aspects of her experience. Angie also reported feeling emotionally blunted and disinterested in activities that previously brought her pleasure. For these reasons, she decided to seek help from a professional in managing her symptoms, particularly her intrusive memories. She stated:

> It got to the point where it became very scary. A memory would pop into my head, and I would be paralyzed. I'd just zone out and stop what I was doing. A couple of times I almost dropped the baby when it happened. I started letting others take care of him, because I was so freaked out when I had these memories. Plus, I just didn't feel connected to him. I didn't seem to care. I knew that I needed to get help or I would risk inadvertently hurting my baby during my "episodes" or would stop acting like his mother altogether.

PTSD is often associated with the same types of life interference and emotional distress discussed in the previous sections. At times, it can disrupt close relationships; for example, it can cause tension in the partner relationship when the woman perceives that her partner does not truly appreciate what she went through or believes that she should "just get over it." As is evident with Angie, posttraumatic stress symptoms stemming from a traumatic childbirth can affect a mother's relationship with her infant. Because the baby serves as a reminder of the trauma, it is possible that new mothers who experienced traumatic childbirths will have intrusive memories of childbirth most often when they are interacting with their babies. A rare and extreme consequence of this vicious cycle is that some mothers might avoid their babies altogether so that they are not reminded of their trauma.

A third consequence of PTSD is numbing: Women report that they have difficulty experiencing any emotions at all. Although, on the surface, numbing may seem adaptive because it protects people from experiencing distressing emotions, it can also deprive new mothers of the joy and satisfaction that can come from parenting a newborn.

PANIC DISORDER

A *panic attack* is a sudden onslaught of anxiety symptoms that seem to come out of nowhere. Although these attacks generally peak within 10 minutes or so, the intense feelings of anxiety can last for an excruciatingly long time, sometimes for hours. These symptoms can include racing heart, difficulty breathing, sweating, shaking, and a sense that one is losing control or going crazy. Between 5 and 10% of the general population report having had a panic attack at some point in their lives (Chen, Tsuchiya, Kawakami, & Furukawa, 2009). A woman is diagnosed with panic disorder when she:

- Is very concerned about having panic attacks in the future
- Worries about the implications or consequences of the panic attack (e.g., that she will have a heart attack)
- Changes her behavior because of the panic attacks

Note that scary thoughts are not part of the definition of panic disorder. Despite this, research has shown that people with panic disorder report one very specific kind of scary thought: the tendency to make catastrophic misinterpretations of bodily sensations (Clark et al., 1997). Consider a situation in which a woman notices that she is a bit short of breath. Some people might attribute shortness of breath to the fact that they just climbed two flights of stairs. Others might notice it but quickly dismiss it, moving on to the next thing that catches their attention.

However, as with Stephanie from Chapter 1, a woman who has the tendency to make catastrophic misinterpretations could attribute that sensation to a malicious "worst-case scenario" outcome, such as lung cancer or some other disease. Moreover, when she makes that interpretation, she has trouble thinking about anything else, and she quickly becomes more and more anxious. In some instances, the cycle of anxiety can become so intense that it spirals out of control and results in a panic attack. The occurrence of frequent panic attacks can lead to even more scary thoughts, such as worry that there must be something terribly wrong, thus creating a vicious cycle.

One consequence of panic disorder is that it can dramatically alter a person's routine. Some people with panic disorder avoid going certain places, like crowded stores, for fear that a panic attack will come out of the blue and that they will be unable to escape. Other people with panic disorder limit their driving because they worry that they will cause an accident if they have a panic attack in traffic. In extreme cases, people with panic disorder do not leave the home for fear of having a panic attack, a condition called *agoraphobia*. It is not difficult to imagine that agoraphobic avoidance would be associated with a great deal of life interference for new mothers, such as avoidance of taking the baby to the park or to the doctor's office.

Agoraphobic avoidance is admittedly an extreme manifestation of panic. But panic attacks that fall anywhere along the continuum can cause dramatic life interference and emotional distress, as with Stephanie. Although her panic attacks did not limit how often she left the house or the activities in which she engaged when she was out and about, her excessive focus on having a terrible lung disease created unnecessary angst. She was alert for the slightest changes in her breathing; if she noticed any hint of difficulty, she began to worry about having lung cancer, which exacerbated her anxiety. She continually sought reassurance from her husband, only to rebuke him when he provided it, claiming that he wasn't a doctor.

These types of interactions frustrated her husband, and he had recently told her that he was at the "end of his rope" and would no longer discuss the subject. This left Stephanie feeling more scared and alone than ever. She wondered if she was going crazy because she could no longer distinguish between changes in her breathing that were to be expected and changes that might signal a problem. She pursued psychotherapy when she was 5 months postpartum in order to develop strategies for managing her anxiety.

REALLY SCARY THOUGHTS

As has been stated previously, the scary thoughts that are the focus of this book are frightening, alarming, and unsettling, but they do not increase the likelihood that a mother will do anything to harm herself or her new baby. They are surprisingly normal occurrences that stem from the combination of genetic, biological, and psychological influences, along with the stress of the transition to parenthood. Although we believe that these kinds of scary thoughts would respond well to most types of psychotherapeutic or pharmacological interventions, providing a woman some much needed relief, professional intervention is not always necessary. In many cases, their frequency diminishes slowly over time. Moreover, many self-help materials can speed up the process of recovery without, or in conjunction with, professional intervention.

Such is not the case for the *really* scary thoughts described in this section. If you or a loved one is experiencing these types of scary thoughts—thoughts that are suicidal or psychotic in nature—then professional intervention is unequivocally indicated. *Really* scary thoughts are associated with an increased likelihood that a mother will harm herself or her child (and, in some cases, older children if they are in the household).

Suicidal Thoughts

A subset of postpartum women in distress may, for the first time in their lives, be faced with agonizing thoughts of despair. When the pain becomes unbearable, some women wonder if the only solution is simply not to be here. Suicidal thoughts (or *suicidal ideation*) are thoughts, images, beliefs, urges, voices, or other cognitions about ending one's life (Wenzel, Brown, & Beck, 2009).

Some suicidal thoughts may be passive (*I wish I could sleep forever and not wake up* or *I wish I were dead*), and some may be active (*I want to hang myself*). Regardless of whether suicidal thoughts are passive or active, it is important to take seriously *any* thoughts of ending one's life. Suicidal ideation is especially concerning when it is accompanied by a desire to die.

Several other factors increase the risk that people who experience suicidal ideation will act on their thoughts: (a) frequency of the thoughts, (b) duration of the thoughts, and (c) intensity of the thoughts. Suicidal thoughts of greater frequency, duration, and intensity are associated with increased risk of making a suicide attempt. If at any time you are having thoughts of suicide, it is important to confide in someone. If you find yourself having these thoughts with increasing frequency, duration, and/or intensity, then this directive becomes all the more important. Tell someone immediately. If you have trouble deciding who to tell, call the National Suicide Prevention Lifeline at 1-800-SUICIDE, where you can talk to someone who will provide you with nonjudgmental support and guidance.

Other types of scary thoughts can accompany suicidal ideation and further increase the risk of making an actual suicide attempt. *Suicidal intent* is the intent to act upon one's suicidal thoughts. Suicidal intent is often accompanied by a plan for the manner in which the suicide attempt will be carried out. These factors increase the risk that a woman will make a suicide attempt because she has set her mind on this decision and may have begun to take steps toward making it happen. Some women experience serious suicidal thoughts when they believe they are a burden to others or if they believe that they do not fit in with the people in their surroundings (Joiner, 2005). These thoughts are scary because they are associated with a sense of hopelessness, loneliness, and emptiness.

Recently, a group of experts on suicide came to a consensus on the warning signs for what they defined as "the earliest detectable sign that indicates heightened risk for suicide in the near-term (i.e., within minutes, hours, or days)" (Rudd et al., 2006, p. 258). They recommended that people call 911 and seek immediate professional help when they or a loved one are threatening to hurt or kill themselves, looking for ways to kill themselves (e.g., seeking out pills or weapons), or talking or writing about killing themselves. Professional help should be sought immediately in these cases because the presence of these warning signs raises the possibility that a person is at imminent risk of harming herself. In addition, the experts recommended that people should seek mental health treatment if they or a loved one:

- Reports hopelessness
- Reports rage or anger
- Acts restless
- Reports feeling trapped
- Increases alcohol or drug use
- Withdraws from others

- Exhibits anxiety or agitation
- Exhibits a dramatic change in mood
- Reports no reason for living or no purpose in life

Although this second group of factors doesn't necessarily mean that a person is acutely suicidal, they create a context for suicidal behavior to emerge when she experiences stress or some sort of adversity.

Many women are reluctant to tell people about their suicidal thoughts because they are worried that they will be sent to the hospital against their will. Although women who are evaluated to be at risk for suicidal behavior are at an increased likelihood of requiring hospitalization, when the risk of harming oneself is not an immediate threat, there are other options. The most effective intervention depends on the particular circumstances, the individual woman, and the healthcare professional's judgment (Wenzel et al., 2009).

Some women decide to see an outpatient therapist, often more than once a week, until the suicidal thoughts subside. Others attend a combination of individual psychotherapy and group psychotherapy. Still others enter what is called partial or day treatment programs. These programs run half or most of the day, 4 or 5 days per week, enabling women to return to their homes in the evening. Some women decide that it is indeed in their best interest to enter an inpatient hospitalization program for a short stay. Healthcare professionals should make every attempt to work collaboratively with a woman who is suffering and her family, taking into account measures to keep her safe, her personal preferences, and her family's circumstances so that the soundest option can be pursued.

Suicidal thoughts are very scary for new mothers. Many mothers who suffer to this degree do not really want to kill themselves. Because they are in so much pain and see no way out of their current situation, they view suicide as the only answer. This is complicated by the fact that their psychological pain has convinced them that their baby, husband, and other family members would be better off without them. Mothers who are suicidal are in a state of sheer desperation. The presence of suicidal thoughts always indicates that professional intervention is required. Fortunately, there is much evidence that suicidal thoughts and the accompanying psychological pain will subside with professional help.

Psychotic Thoughts

Psychotic thoughts are *really* scary thoughts that, in postpartum women, are sometimes associated with aggressive urges to do serious harm to themselves or others, usually the newborn. On the surface, they may seem similar to obsessive thoughts about intentionally inflicting harm upon the new baby. However, the two are actually quite different. As stated in Chapter 2, obsessive thoughts are ego-dystonic, which means that they are inconsistent with what a woman believes to be true and cause a great deal of alarm and distress. In sharp contrast, psychotic thoughts are *ego-syntonic,* which means that they make logical sense to those who experience them and do not cause distress or alarm.

In other words, women who experience obsessive thoughts still think and behave like themselves, despite intermittent thoughts about harming the baby that are extremely frightening. Women who experience psychotic thoughts temporarily exist in a distorted reality in which thoughts of harming the baby often play a central role. Within her distorted sense of reality, a mother may show no signs of distress because her bizarre thinking feels real to her. This is why it is crucial that she get immediate professional help in order to treat this psychotic state.

If you are having scary thoughts about harming your baby, you may be frantically wondering if your thoughts are psychotic in nature. The mere fact that you are frightened and concerned about your thoughts suggests that they are obsessive thoughts, not psychotic thoughts. Remember that obsessive thoughts are very common, occurring in up to 91% of new mothers. Psychotic thoughts, in contrast, are very *un*common, occurring in only one or two of every thousand postpartum women (Kendall, Chalmers, & Platz, 1987). In some cases, they develop suddenly after delivery, often around 3 weeks following childbirth (Brockington et al., 1981), but there are cases when they are detected later in the postpartum period. Furthermore, psychotic thoughts are most likely to occur in women who have a history of serious mental illness, especially bipolar disorder (Jones & Craddock, 2001).

If you are still having trouble differentiating between obsessive thoughts about harming your baby and psychotic thoughts, it may be helpful to consider some of the other features of postpartum psychosis. Symptoms that often accompany postpartum psychosis include extreme agitation, confusion, exhilaration, extreme mood lability, and an inability to sleep or eat (Beck & Driscoll, 2006). Others will notice that your behavior is much different from your usual behavior and may have difficulty holding a coherent conversation with you. You might be experiencing hallucinations, when you see or hear things that are not really there. All of these symptoms are serious and suggest that you are having trouble maintaining an accurate sense of reality.

The presence of psychotic thoughts is an emergency that needs to be treated aggressively and always requires hospitalization. It is understandable that most women would find the prospect of staying at a hospital terribly frightening. However, there are several benefits of hospitalization. First and foremost, it will provide a safe environment that will prevent harm coming to you and your baby. Second, healthcare providers will be able to start you on medications that will reduce your symptoms. Oftentimes, you will be started on more than one medication in order to stabilize your mood more quickly and to decrease your psychotic thinking (Beck & Driscoll, 2006). Third, hospitalization allows for a treatment plan to be put in place that will provide you the support and professional help you will need as you transition back to caring for your child in your home. Although postpartum psychosis is undoubtedly alarming and confusing for you and your family, there is every indication that with proper treatment you will recover in a timely manner (Platz & Kendall, 1988).

MOVING FORWARD

The psychiatric diagnoses described in this chapter provide a clinical context for scary thoughts. Some women find comfort in knowing there is a name that corresponds to their scary thoughts and emotional experience. Other women do not care one way or another—they just want relief. Still other women find the notion of psychiatric diagnoses to be disconcerting. The most important point is that a woman can address her scary thoughts according to whatever framework is most helpful to her.

If the diagnostic context is overwhelming or unsettling to you, disregard this chapter and move on to one that feels more helpful or more relevant to your experience. Remember that, even if it seems as if you might meet criteria for one of these diagnoses, a healthcare provider should confirm this. Ideally, it is preferable that you consult with a professional who specializes in postpartum anxiety and mood disorders; however, if you are not able to find a specialist, consulting with a mental health practitioner with whom you feel safe is an excellent option. Regardless of whether or not you have a psychiatric diagnosis or whether or not you choose to understand your scary thoughts in the context of a psychiatric diagnosis, the remainder of this book will provide information and strategies that should help you to get relief from your distress and put these thoughts in perspective.

Take-Home Point for Mothers. Each of the types of scary thoughts described in this book is associated with a psychiatric diagnosis. If you suspect that you meet criteria for one of these diagnoses, it will be important to confirm this with a healthcare provider. There are well established psychotherapeutic and pharmacological interventions that can treat these conditions. Even if you don't think you meet criteria for a psychiatric disorder, you can still experience scary thoughts, and you still may want to seek treatment for them. The most important factors to consider are whether the scary thoughts are causing interference in your life and/or whether they are distressing for you.

Clinician Note. If a postpartum woman reports scary thoughts, it will be important to assess for the presence of the anxiety and mood disorders described in this chapter, understanding that such a diagnosis might be met with denial, resistance, or even relief. In order to determine the appropriate level of care, be sure to evaluate her level of emotional distress regarding her scary thoughts, as well as perform a comprehensive suicide risk assessment.

5

Barriers to Relief

Every time Liza put her 4-month-old baby in his car seat, she had visions of him sliding out of the seat (after being carefully strapped in), somehow being hurled out the car window (though it was winter and all the windows were shut), and his little body splattering onto the roadway. It didn't stop her from driving, but it often kept her from making trips alone with the baby if she had to drive far. When her husband told her she was being ridiculous for worrying so much about driving, she decided to tell him exactly what she was afraid of and shared the details of her private thoughts. Hoping for a reprieve, Liza sank further when her husband agreed that driving the baby was not a good idea. After all, if she was afraid the baby would fall out of the car, then she shouldn't have the baby in the car with her. He continued to ramble on about her questionable driving skill. Liza stopped listening right about the time he said he would get his mother to take the baby to all future doctor appointments.

That's when she stopped telling her husband what she was thinking.

The literature supports this anecdote, in that women with postpartum distress are reluctant to make their negative feelings known to others. One study found that five out of six women with postpartum depression were hesitant to reveal their symptoms, ultimately delaying treatment and recovery. These women believed that their symptoms reflected their inability to cope as mothers and feared that their babies would be taken away from them if they exposed how they felt (Edwards & Timmons, 2005). There are lots of reasons why new mothers don't talk about the thoughts they are having, particularly the scary ones. People don't like talking about things that make them feel bad. This is true in general. But for a woman who is inundated by expectations that she should glide into the role of mother effortlessly and without protest, this notion of expressing anything negative about the experience can feel irreverent, almost sacrilegious.

Postpartum women who experience scary thoughts have a sense of trepidation about themselves as well as the people around them. They can't possibly imagine how anyone could understand or accept such abomination. It doesn't matter how chilling or how innocuous the thought may be; a mother who experiences it plunges right into a dark and unforgiving hole. For many, the leap from thinking they could slip and drop their baby down the stairs is only a heartbeat away from fear that they might drown the baby in the bathtub or stab the baby with a kitchen knife. As a result of this profound agitation, it is common for these women to submit to their private pain and detach themselves from those who may be in the best position to help them. We have seen how the conflict of feeling such great love and coexisting horror can drive some women deeper into isolation.

WHY WOMEN DON'T TELL

It is well documented that postpartum women are reluctant to share the fact that they are anxious or depressed. In one study that investigated feelings, patterns of help-seeking behaviors, and treatment options associated with postpartum depression, 90% of women in the sample said that they knew something was wrong, but only one third of them believed they had postpartum depression. Furthermore, over 80% stated they had not reported their symptoms to any healthcare professional (Whitton, Warner, & Appleby, 1996). Myriad factors contribute to a woman's reluctance to put words to the thoughts that are scaring her. As you consider the following obstacles, bear in mind those factors that relate to your situation so that you can refer back to them when you record your notes in Chapter 11.

The Ambiguity Factor: What's Really Going On Here?

As Karen points out in her book, *Therapy and the Postpartum Woman* (Kleiman, 2008), perhaps the foremost reason why postpartum anxiety and depression are frequently misdiagnosed is the ambiguity of symptoms.

This is due to the overlapping experiences between women with postpartum anxiety or depression and women with no such diagnosis. For example, fatigue, loss of libido, moodiness, weepiness, changes in weight, sleep disturbance, and low energy can all be attributed to anxiety and depression, yet they are also considered to be within normal expectations for postpartum adjustment (Kleiman, 2008; Yonkers, 1995). Considering the fact that healthcare professionals are sometimes perplexed when determining which experiences are problematic and which are not, how can we really expect postpartum women to make this determination with accuracy? As we discussed earlier in the book, postpartum women often do not know when they might need help.

Postpartum women often express sweeping uncertainties regarding how they are feeling. Because moods and other internal experiences are expected to fluctuate following childbirth, women sometimes decide it is best to brave any discomfort and hope it goes away by itself. Unfortunately, scary thoughts are not easy to ride out. What's more, without proper assessment, a woman's worry about these thoughts can rapidly disintegrate from initial concern to panic.

The Critical Inner Voice: How You Feel About Yourself and Your Thoughts

The shame that can accompany upsetting thoughts is unbearable. *What is wrong with me? How can I be thinking these things? Good mothers don't think such terrible thoughts.* Often, the only explanation that makes sense to a mother who is trying to reconcile this disturbing experience is that there is something profoundly wrong with her, that something is broken inside. Maybe she is close to insanity. Or maybe she is not fit to be a mother. Either option, or anything in between, is a nightmare. This nightmare stuns many women into silence. They hope that if they can just hold their breath and carry off this role-play, their awful thoughts will somehow go away. In some instances, the thoughts actually do go away. Usually, they do not.

Other women tirelessly try to push the thoughts out of their minds, but are distraught when the thoughts return in full force. Recall Lori from Chapter 1. Karen asked her if she felt comfortable sharing the scary thoughts she was having. Lori sat with her head down, gasping with shallow breaths as she spoke, "I can't tell you what I'm thinking. I can't. I'm a disgusting person. I can hardly stand myself. Something is seriously wrong. You have to help me." It can be difficult for a clinician to sit back and listen to the scathing, self-loathing words springing from the lips of a mother in pain. "Stop it. Stop it. Stop it," Lori cried anxiously as she pressed her fingers into her forehead in a futile effort to stifle the noise in her head. "Seriously, how can I think what I'm thinking. It's revolting. *I'm* revolting."

Some women can express the horror of their thoughts along with the abysmal shame that accompanies them, but, for many, the actual articulation of the specific thoughts—the words they fear would somehow make the thoughts come alive—remains locked inside. When women feel they are in a safe place, they are more apt to reveal the nature of some of their scary thoughts. Despite this, the actual expression of the precise thought or image itself can still remain buried beneath the remorse and remain unsaid, often for very long periods of time.

In other words, even when women are in a safe setting and divulge some aspects of their scary thoughts, they may continue to hide other aspects or reveal some thoughts but not others. Women say they are embarrassed, ashamed, mortified, humiliated, and guilty beyond description. They say they feel hideously exposed, naked, repulsive, raw, nauseous, ugly, and sickened by their own thoughts. Some say they feel so appalled by the nature of their thoughts that they feel inhuman, as if only a monster could possess and admit such atrocities.

In Chapter 2, we discussed that this high level of distress indicates that the thoughts are ego-dystonic—incompatible with the woman's sense of herself. It bears repeating that, although it is never easy to experience or witness such high levels of distress, there is considerably more concern when a woman expresses no such distress or displays no strong affect attached to this worry. Thus, even though the presentation can be overwhelming, it also serves as a signal that anxiety is the mechanism at work and not something more worrisome, like psychosis. Knowing this can reassure both the distressed mother and the healthcare provider.

Shame-based barriers to a mother's disclosing her thoughts can be fueled by the critic inside her head. With regard to the critical inner voice, mothers tell us they are reluctant to reveal scary thoughts because they:

- Fear that they are the only mother who has ever felt this way and that no one could possibly understand

- Believe that the thoughts they are having are an indication that something is terribly wrong
- Worry that, if they admit this, they will indeed be crazy
- Worry that they will be locked up or institutionalized
- Fear that saying it out loud will make the bad thought a reality
- Believe that good mothers don't think these thoughts
- Hate themselves for having the thoughts and remain stifled by intense shame and guilt
- May not be comfortable talking about how they feel, in general

Everyone has an inner voice. This voice can guide people through difficult times with reason and good judgment, or it can cut into someone's best efforts by viciously condemning each step. In this way, a person's self-esteem is closely linked to her relationship with her own inner critic. Consider this ordinary circumstance in which a woman finds herself in a situation that triggers her inner voice: *I wonder if I need to go help my friend with her project after work. She did say we could meet next week, and I really should get home to make dinner. But we made these plans weeks ago and I told her I would …*

Someone with solid self-esteem might decide that it's fine to postpone the plans to get together, extend her apologies, and reschedule for another day. In contrast, someone with lower self-esteem may mull this over with anxiety and guilt, worrying that her friend will be mad if she cancels. But if she goes, she'll resent her friend, and her kids will have to wait for dinner or eat fish sticks again. Either way, she loses ground. At The Postpartum Stress Center, this type of circular reflection is affectionately referred to as the "I-suck" tape that loops perpetually in a woman's head, making it impossible to think clearly. Women who find themselves stuck worrying, ruminating, or obsessing often default to thinking how much they suck and are unable to see or think their way out.

Strong self-esteem enables women to quiet the chatter from their critical inner voice. Conversely, learning to turn down the volume of the critical voice will strengthen self-esteem. When women are weakened by childbirth, the demands of the postpartum period, or anxious or depressive symptoms, they are easily wounded and defenseless against the attacks of the inner critic. This is when excessive worry, rumination, obsessive thinking, intrusive memories, and catastrophic misinterpretation of bodily symptoms are likely to emerge.

The paradox is this: The critical inner voice must be disarmed in order to maintain power. When they are most vulnerable, women believe this voice to be invincible. In truth, this voice only has as much power as women give it.

The Sentencing: What Others Will Think of You

Liza, the mother of the 4-month-old mentioned earlier in this chapter, discovered that after she shared some of her thoughts with her unmarried girlfriend, her friend spent less and less time with her. Liza reflected on this: "I think I made her nervous. Either she thought I was crazy or she just didn't know how to be with me. I guess if it's hard for her to be my friend, I'd rather find that out now."

Many women say they are extremely apprehensive about being labeled or diagnosed as mentally ill. Although it's true that a number of women diagnosed with postpartum anxiety or depression express relief in knowing that it is a real medical condition that is treatable, most continue to feel burdened by what others might think. Thus, any diagnosis attached to motherhood presents as an oxymoron of sorts; it weighs heavily on the heart of a mother trying to do her best and impedes postpartum healing.

A few years ago, Karen distributed an informal questionnaire at The Postpartum Stress Center, asking women to whom they were most likely to report symptoms of postpartum anxiety and depression prior to seeking treatment at the center. She and her staff were seeking to determine patterns of behavior that would help maximize successful paths of reporting and treatment. The tendency to remain silent for long periods was impressive. The majority of the women reported they were most comfortable first telling someone in their family rather than in the medical community. Most indicated that their husbands and/or mothers were the first line of admitting to symptoms, but even that was only after an extended period of suffering. Regarding their healthcare providers, the women unequivocally indicated that they would first tell their obstetrician and not report symptoms to their pediatrician.

Although we discuss screening practices with healthcare professionals in the following chapter, it's important to make a couple of notes here regarding disclosure to these individuals. The women who responded to the survey felt strongly about their preference to talk with their obstetrician because they (a) felt more comfortable discussing feelings with this particular healthcare professional, indicating a level of intimacy that accompanies the pregnancy and childbirth experience; and (b) believed that symptoms related to the postpartum period fell within the confines of the obstetrical specialty.

Their reasons for not talking to their pediatrician were varied, but all centered on one theme. Women were most fearful of being judged by the baby's doctor or perceived as unfit to be a mother. Their responses ranged from anxiety that the pediatrician would disapprove of their mothering tendencies to the irrational fear that the baby would be taken away from them. Many of the mothers who responded to this survey confessed they went to great lengths to create the impression that they were feeling fine, particularly in the presence of their baby's doctor.

We also see this dynamic burst forth in social settings, particularly in the company of other mothers, where the temptation to judge and feel judged can run rampant. One young mother referred to this as the "playground imperative" because it seemed to her to be a universal and inevitable postpartum experience. Women find themselves in the presence of that nameless perfect mother at the playground (or anywhere else), who interacts with her perfect children and seems to meet every single unattainable expectation. She looks flawless from head to toe and says and does all the right things. We've all seen her. Every new mother reports the occasional pang of self-rejection and the deafening ring of the *I-suck* tape.

Along with what others may think is a woman's concern about the impact her disclosure will have on someone close to her. For example, women say they are hesitant to tell their partners how bad they are feeling or the specific nature of their thoughts because they don't want their partners to worry more about them or become fearful concerning their or their babies' well-being. Some women state they fear their husbands will overreact and that this additional worry will add an extra thick layer of anxiety on top of what they already endure on their own.

Common barriers related to what others might think include women:

- Worrying that someone will judge them
- Worrying that someone will label them as bad mothers
- Worrying that someone will take their baby away

- Worrying that their partner or family will deem them incapable of taking care of the baby
- Thinking that a healthcare provider doesn't want to know or can't help or not trusting the healthcare provider to understand and respond appropriately
- Not seeing mental health issues as part of their provider's job description
- Having concerns about confidentiality and what may happen if they reveal what they are thinking

What others think can have more influence over how women feel and ultimately act than they care to admit. The bottom line here is that if mothers are not careful, this propensity to condemn their thoughts or behavior in some way shifts the authority of these thoughts in the wrong direction, thereafter empowering the thoughts even more. This is another example of the manner in which faulty thinking leads to excessive worry and impairs access to recovery. Women need to speak on their own behalf, trust their inclinations to reach out for support, and worry less about what misinformed friends or acquaintances might think.

The Depression Factor: What You May Be Thinking Because of How You Feel

Women with depression think negatively. Some theorize that biological factors influence negative thinking, which can lead to depression. Others claim that pessimistic or negative thought processes can contribute to the emergence of depression. Though this question of biology versus cognition in depression is up for debate, experts agree that a significant correlation exists between the two. When thoughts are distorted, perceptions become darker, scarier, and magnified out of proportion. Nerves are exposed, leaving women feeling hypersensitive and thin skinned. This feeling of overexposure can create a sense of mistrust in the outside world; women can grow suspicious of how others might respond to knowing the "truth" about what they were thinking and feeling.

Symptoms of depression also thwart a woman's desire to seek help by immobilizing her. She's exhausted. She's frightened. Or, she simply doesn't care enough right now. Feelings of despair, fatigue, and apathy may have set in. She may simply feel too tired to make the phone call or drive to an appointment. She may be hoping it will all go away on its own. She may find it difficult to focus or concentrate on the things she needs to do. What she may not realize yet is that, as she recovers from the depressive symptoms, she will begin to think more clearly. In the meantime, women with depressive symptoms may need to push through the inertia and reach out for help, despite the temptation to remain still within their pain. Mobilizing the body and spirit against the weight of depression is surely easier to suggest than it is to do.

Wendy was 6 weeks postpartum when she described her hesitation to talk with her doctor:

> I sat waiting in the cold room, wrapped in the peach-colored gown tied loosely in the front, wondering whether I should let my doctor know how much I was freaking myself out. I remember feeling freezing and nervous, rocking my body back and forth while my shaking legs dangled over the exam table. After what felt like forever, my doctor walked in with a smile and said something like, "So, you feeling good?" Close to losing my nerve, I was quick to say, "No." There was no turning back. Did she hear me? Would she want me to elaborate? I watched the doctor dutifully fill out some lab sheets and peruse my patient file. She must not have heard me. Why wasn't she saying anything? Maybe she thought I was kidding. I waited and sighed heavily. My doctor turned and looked at my face, which was probably as white as a ghost: "Is there something you want to tell me about the way you are feeling?" I think so, I answered silently inside my head ... I think so.

Depression is a self-absorbing illness. It can rob you of your desire to seek appropriate care and can interfere with any effort even to try. Depressive thinking can inhibit your attempts to deal appropriately with your scary thoughts by distorting or exaggerating the possible outcomes of disclosing. Making a good decision on your own behalf is stymied when everything is perceived through the lens of depressive thinking.

The Propaganda Factor: Sorting Through the Half-Truths

Tons of misunderstandings and misperceptions surround this phenomenon of scary thoughts during motherhood. As previously pointed out, this lack of knowledge spans from woman to woman, to healthcare professionals, and to society as a whole. Without widespread consensus on whether a situation signals immediate danger or is a transient state of acute anxiety, women will continue to question where they fall along that continuum.

Moreover, each woman is indeed unique, with her own history, set of circumstances, personal experiences, and interpretations that must be taken into consideration.

Postpartum women frequently find themselves at the mercy of well-meaning, but often misinformed, family and friends, who can be incredible sources of support, but who can also unwittingly sabotage a mother's recovery with false information. In addition, dedicated healthcare professionals are not always correctly informed and can react in ways that cause further difficulties for a struggling mother. In desperation, many women find themselves seeking answers from the countless anonymous advisers in cyberspace who may not hesitate to promote their own explanations for what may or may not be going on. It is generally recommended that postpartum women steer clear of the Internet as a sole source of support until they have ample understanding of what they are experiencing and what, if anything, they need to do about it. We discuss the advantages and disadvantages of seeking online support in Chapter 7.

As we write this book, both of us recall numerous women who came to us for support, panicked after reading some bit of drama on the Internet that someone had spun in the wrong direction. Lori came into Karen's office telling her that earlier that day she had read a blurb about anxiety after childbirth; it ended with a disclaimer that said something like, "If you're having any thoughts that are frightening you, it is always an extreme emergency. If you cannot get yourself to the emergency room, call 911 right now." Then, in capital letters, it read: "DO NOT UNDER ANY CIRCUMSTANCES STAY ALONE WITH YOUR BABY!" By the time she got to her session, her heart was racing, and her pulse was high. She was close to hyperventilating, and she wondered if she had made a mistake by bringing the baby with her, or if she should have driven straight to the hospital.

Lori was fine, but she was in a fragile state and susceptible to the pangs of misleading and unfounded messages. She needed accurate information, clarification, support, reassurance, and a comprehensive evaluation from someone knowledgeable in this field. Because Lori was already receiving treatment, she had a safe place to unload her anxiety and regain perspective, but it is easy to see how so many women could feel paralyzed by reading such sweeping statements. Generalizations that are splashed in print or other media outlets may not be pertinent to a mother who is suffering, or they may be totally irrelevant or erroneous. Internalizing more negative information can reinforce the inherent resistance to seek help. It is best for women not to place too much emphasis on unsubstantiated statements and always to check out the sources of information that may lead to potential agitation.

The Community Factor: Support and Stigma

Communities can hold great power—the power to heal as well as the power to discriminate. Within all communities, we see the interplay of social support, the stigma of mental illness, and a variety of cultural influences. Postpartum women, who rely heavily on the support of others for comfort and healing, must wade through their own notions of what mothers should and should not feel or think and that which is expected from within a community context (e.g., idealized expectations that a mother be strong or perfect, return to work immediately, or stay home indefinitely).

The stigma of mental illness is pervasive. It remains steadfast, in spite of current wisdom and widespread attempts to inform and enlighten women and healthcare providers across cultures. Although we must be alert to specific cultural expectations that can impose high standards for mothers to meet, we cannot ignore the research literature, which consistently demonstrates that communities with strong social support provide shelter and yield lower rates of postpartum depression (O'Hara, 1995). This dichotomy can send mixed messages to the mother who is trying to juggle her desire to comply with expectations from all directions. The message to a new mother should be for her to prioritize her social support, regardless of the pressure she feels from either a perceived stigma or cultural mandate.

Research has demonstrated that social support helps to alleviate symptoms of depression and hastens recovery (O'Hara & Swain, 1996). However, if social stigma precludes a woman's asking for help or prevents the person or person in whom she confides from receiving or accepting what is being disclosed, there is an impasse. If she is afraid she will be chastised, she will shrink back into isolation. There is a general tendency for women to recoil from social support when they feel judged or stigmatized; this is true across cultures. Regardless of cultural practices, the intrinsic value of acceptance and support within family and community networks presents as a recurring theme that can either encourage or hinder recovery (Knudson-Martin & Silverstein, 2009).

An in-depth examination of the social rituals and expectations of different cultures is beyond the scope of this book, although we explore social support in greater detail in Chapter 10. Nevertheless, the impact of various practices is crucial to consider when exploring why women continue to be silenced by the fear of their own thoughts in addition to the fear of how their community will respond to these thoughts. Although the work referenced next specifically targets the population of women with postpartum depression, we believe strongly that women with symptoms of anxiety or scary thoughts struggle similarly, whether or not they have been assigned a diagnosis.

A comprehensive analysis of postpartum depression revealed the manner in which the despair of depression can isolate women who feel pressured by cultural standards (Knudson-Martin & Silverstein, 2009). The authors of this study cited several individual studies, whose results demonstrate that significant cultural influences are at work in determining whether women will disclose their thoughts. This work revealed an array of culture-specific taboos that resonate with postpartum women and contribute to their isolation.

For example, African American women reported perceiving a strong need to comply with expectations that they be survivors by "wearing the mask" (Amankwaa, 2003). One Chinese woman stated that, after she had her baby, she felt as if she lost control over her emotions and ability to cope, failing to measure up to her idealized concept of motherhood. Some Chinese women reported "phantom crying." Although it is common for postpartum women to wake during the night and check on their baby, this auditory phenomenon refers to actually hearing the baby cry when he is not crying. Such an experience can occur with extreme anxiety (Chan, Levy, Chung, & Lee, 2002). British women reported wrestling with perceived expectations of perfection (Mauthner, 2002).

Because of this steadfast cultural expectation for mothers to achieve and exude precise control, a woman who looks to her family, friends, and healthcare providers might find this message reinforced with words or references to disappointment—for example: *I'm surprised you need help with the baby. I didn't need help with two!* Remarks such as this can quickly silence the voice of the suffering mother. Thus, various cultural taboos surrounding the challenges of motherhood appear to be sustained by a society at large and also perpetuated by women themselves (Mauthner, 2002). Either way, we see how important it is to establish a social context in which mothers can feel free to express both positive and negative feelings and thoughts related to their mothering experience.

Oftentimes, family and social responses to help-seeking behaviors are also culture-specific. Deciding to seek professional help can be difficult, but it will be further complicated if a woman anticipates or perceives disapproval of this decision. Lack of emotional and practical support must be addressed because it continues to be the subject of universal disappointment expressed by postpartum women. Although many women report to us that they are profoundly grateful for the support that they receive, they simultaneously see this support as insufficient.

In many cases, women claim that, despite ongoing and abundant support, the expectation to express only positive feelings attached to the mothering experience remains high. The tendency for women with acute distress to suffer in silence persists, reinforcing the concern that social support systems, though crucial to postpartum healing, remain inadequate to some extent. Perhaps the greatest menace is the inability to accept the presence of negative thoughts and feelings during this time. Only when this takes place can postpartum women be expected to speak from their hearts and break through their reluctance to disclose.

The "What If" Factor: What Actions Might Result From Disclosure?

The best way to summarize the anxiety-drenched roadblocks to disclosure of scary thoughts is to view them in terms of "what ifs." As we've seen throughout this chapter, withholding can be attributable to countless factors: A woman is ambivalent or unclear about what she is thinking, her inner critic is negative and boisterous, she believes she is being unduly judged by those around her, she believes all the unjustified things she reads, and she wonders if she will be ostracized from her family of origin for thinking this way. All or any of these barriers culminates to create this ultimate deterrent: What if something bad happens as a result of my disclosure?

In 2007, a journalist for the *Star-Ledger* (Newark, New Jersey) reported on a case that demonstrates what can happen when misinformed healthcare practitioners overreact to scary thoughts. After one woman confided in her gynecologist about scary thoughts involving the violent death of her baby, she was escorted from the office to the emergency room by a policeman and social worker (Livio, 2007). This illustrates a mother's worst fear: that if she reveals these deep dark thoughts, she will be whisked away into oblivion.

Katherine Stone, author of "Postpartum Progress," the most widely read blog on postpartum depression and anxiety, describes her own anxiety and the fear of her anxiety during her struggle with acute postpartum anxiety and scary thoughts:

> ... And the thought came into my head, what if I drown him in the bathtub? That was the end of bath-giving. I don't believe I gave my son another bath for at least a year. I told my husband that he'd have to do it ... And it wasn't like voices; nobody was telling me to do anything. It was simply that a thought that I didn't purposefully generate came into my head. How do you explain to someone you are not the thinker of the thoughts? But it's your thoughts. I was sure if I said that, the paddy wagon would show up at my front door and I'd never see my family again, I mean I was convinced. So I didn't tell anyone exactly what I was thinking. (http://postpartumprogress.typepad.com)

When a woman is in or expects to be in a potentially anxiety-provoking situation, such as disclosing her scary thoughts, she might respond by focusing on imaginary dangers. This is referred to as anticipatory anxiety, which is typically characterized by *what-if* thinking patterns. For example, women with panic disorder might worry about having a panic attack in a situation that might result in embarrassment or shame (*What if I feel like I can't breathe and start to panic when I'm in the store and totally feel like I will lose control?*) Even women without a diagnosis of panic disorder can be very familiar with "what if" worries. They are virtually infectious during the postpartum period.

Women in our clinical practices concur that the list of anxious *what-if* worries is endless. The assortment of *what ifs* crosses the boundaries of all the barriers to disclosure. That is, no matter why a woman is hesitant to reveal what she is thinking, she is sure to include a few *what ifs* in her anxiety-driven expressions:

- What if they take my baby away?
- What if they call child protection services?
- What if they think I'm a bad mother?
- What if they don't like me?
- What if they think I'm crazy?
- What if they put me in a hospital?
- What if they think I could really hurt my baby?

- What if I really do hurt my baby?
- What if this means I really AM crazy?
- What if my husband leaves me?
- What if I never get better?
- What if I can't really trust this person?
- What if they can't help me?
- What if they can help me, but I am labeled for life?
- What if my friends or neighbors find out (and think I'm crazy)?
- What if my mom (parents, family) think I am not a good mother?
- What if someone at my other children's school finds out, and this affects my other children?
- What if people at work find out, and it affects my career?
- What if letting someone know how I feel makes it more real somehow?
- What if I will always feel and think this way?

Imagine if we put all of this anxiety to good use. It is possible, conversely, to have a list of *what ifs* with a positive spin:

- What if I talk about what I'm thinking, and I get the help I need?
- What if my husband (family, friend, doctor) reassures me, and I am comforted by my decision to talk about this?
- What if, by talking about this, I get relief, and I feel less guilty?
- What if talking about it frees me up to make room for other feelings, such as joy or serenity?
- What if I trust myself and the people around me and take a leap of faith that I will get help or reassurance?
- What if I discover that what I am feeling and thinking is not so bizarre and that lots of other women feel this way?
- What if it's true that the way I am feeling is a common response to motherhood?
- What if I believe this can and will get better?

Generally speaking, it appears that postpartum women appreciate being able to talk to a sympathetic and supportive listener who allows them to express their fears and unburden themselves. Intervention at this level rests with efforts to increase awareness of their irrational fears, while establishing a context in which women can feel safe to express what they think and feel. Once this begins, women will learn to feel more confident about the process and will be better equipped to restructure some of their thinking patterns.

HEALTHCARE PROVIDER BARRIERS

We've seen how fear-induced resistance can obstruct a mother's path to healing. The other side of this issue is that, despite an increase in public awareness, healthcare providers inadvertently contribute to the perpetuation of this gridlock. Providers often do not ask the right questions or are reticent to ask the questions at all. Worse yet, in the absence of knowledgeable alternatives, they hand out pills and platitudes. Still, even when a provider asks the right questions, women often respond tentatively and may not disclose the extent to which they are suffering. Thus, we have attempts that go nowhere, reinforced by miscommunication on both sides.

Healthcare providers may fail to ask whether a mother is having scary thoughts because they:

- Are misinformed
- Are unaware of how common this phenomenon is with all women who give birth, not just those with a diagnosis of postpartum anxiety disorders or depression
- Mistakenly presume that scary thoughts are associated with only severe illnesses and reserve that question for women who present with more complex clinical pictures
- Are unsure of how to proceed if they get a positive response
- Lack sufficient information and skill sets to intervene appropriately
- Have limited time with each patient
- Focus solely on how she is recovering physically from childbirth
- May not consider it to be a crucial component of their routine screening procedures
- May be deceived by how good and healthy a patient looks
- Hesitate to raise mental health-related concerns if they are not mental health experts
- Have their own mental health issues and are reluctant to address such issues with their patients

- May not believe they have established a close enough relationship with the woman
- See it as someone else's responsibility

As new studies reveal a strong biological component to postpartum changes and illnesses, experts are hopeful that this will help eliminate the stigma associated with negative feelings, thoughts, or images after childbirth. If even healthy brains are wired to experience some degree of anxiety, it should not surprise us that these feelings are intensified during vulnerable periods. As more is learned about the function of the brain, healthcare providers can offset strong emotional responses by offering more information and support. In the next chapter, we will address screening and clinical practices and explore how best to facilitate good communication between the postpartum woman and those who are in a position to care for her.

As we've seen, feelings associated with normal postpartum adjustment, as well as those linked with postpartum anxiety or depression, can lead to deep shame and isolation. It is essential that spouses, family members, friends, and healthcare professionals learn to listen to and tolerate these feelings. Only then will women feel secure enough to engage in the open dialogue that needs to take place and be able to trust the outcome.

Take-Home Point for Mothers. Although it is understandable that your fears would interfere with your ability to disclose how you are feeling, sometimes trust in yourself and in your relationships can be the ultimate remedy. Do not surrender to the temptation to remain silent. You will feel better if you share the burden of your pain with someone you trust.

Clinician Note. Understanding the unique nature of a postpartum woman's resistance to disclose will enable you to access the empathy required to facilitate healing. You are obliged to honor this resistance, while at the same time being careful not to reinforce her inclination to isolate and withhold.

6

Screening for Scary Thoughts

I told no one, except my husband knew obviously that I was depressed, but my sisters came down for Christmas and all the while I'm having scary thoughts that I'm going to hurt my baby and I don't want to see anyone and I'm terrified all the time. I would put a Santa suit on the baby and they would think I was just fine.

Mary Jo Codey

Former First Lady of New Jersey (Mededppd.org)

How does a woman move forward when her deeply rooted fears keep her from telling the truth to those who surround her with love and support? How does she confide in others in the face of such widespread misunderstanding and potential for alarm? We have discussed various barriers to disclosure and subsequent relief from the woman's standpoint—the overlap of normal postpartum worries and those that are problematic, thinking and feeling badly about herself, the perception that others will think negatively of her, overreaction to misleading information, rigid social and cultural expectations, and the overwhelmingly pervasive fear that any disclosure is bound to lead to something catastrophic. But a postpartum woman's unwillingness to reveal the extent to which she is suffering, in general, and the nature of her scary thoughts, in particular, is still only half the problem.

Women in distress can only be expected to feel as comfortable as their environment enables, thus underscoring the role of the healthcare providers who are in a position to help. Much of the content of this chapter is applicable to clinical settings where screening practices are conducted. The reason we have included this information within the heart of this book is to empower postpartum women further by furnishing them with accurate information they can utilize within the context of their own experiences. We hope that you will be able to take what you've learned here into your doctor's office and facilitate a clearer dialogue about how you are feeling and what you may need.

In this chapter, we take a closer look at some of the screening practices that should ideally take place and the factors that might facilitate or sabotage these efforts. You may notice that the tone of this chapter leans toward the clinician, as we aspire to guide providers in their effort to maximize available resources on behalf of postpartum women. Again, this is a case in which we feel strongly that although the healthcare provider and the postpartum woman may have different agendas, they are both seeking similar outcomes and can benefit from enhanced awareness.

AWARENESS

In healthcare or clinical settings where women are presumably in the care of providers who are well equipped to provide relief, women who harbor scary thoughts remain reluctant to reveal what they are thinking. When women are asked specifically if they are having scary thoughts, they might respond in a number of different ways, depending on who is asking, how the person asks it, why the person asks, and what the mother has to gain or lose by answering. Because of these variables, we should first consider a mother's personal experience in the context of being directly asked about the scary thoughts she may not have come to terms with having in the first place. After all, we've seen that what is scary for one person may not feel scary to another. This is illustrated by the array of responses that provide insight into the vast range of interpretations of questions about scary thoughts.

At The Postpartum Stress Center, during an initial phone intake, clinicians ask: *Are you having any thoughts that are scaring you?* When this question regarding scary thoughts is asked, it is deliberately left open ended to encourage an individual interpretation. The following are commonly heard responses to the question, *Are you having any thoughts that are scaring you?*

Silence. This response can mean a number of things, ranging from taking time to think, to a pause for clarification, to a quiet panic, or hesitation to disclose. It is reasonable that the caller would be wary of the question or the person on the other end of the phone asking the question. Clearly, the phone is not the best medium for self-disclosure of this nature; however, given the potential crisis inherent in working with postpartum women, it is often the first line of intervention.

Oh, no. I don't want to hurt my baby or anything like that. I love my baby. Many women immediately flash to the sensationalism put forth by misleading media attention and think the question is trying to scope out whether there is intent to harm the baby. The truth is, whether there is intent to harm the baby or not, most women will not reveal this on the phone. Whether or not the answer is truthful at this early stage is less relevant than the fact that she knows she is speaking with someone who understands that scary thoughts can be a part of her current experience.

Yes. I'm scared I'm not going to feel better. Although some women presume that scary thoughts pertain only to thoughts of harm coming to the baby, as we've seen, any thought can be scary if it is experienced as such. It can certainly feel scary to think that one will always feel this bad. This response demonstrates the ruminative quality of some postpartum thought processes, which may or may not indicate that there are additional scary thoughts lurking.

Well, sometimes it scares me that something bad could happen, like I could snap and do something terrible. This response reveals the woman's initial trust in the dialogue and her willingness to reach out for help. This is an instance in which further probing, done in a sensitive manner, would be appropriate to determine if emergency intervention is necessary or if reassurance and an appointment would be appropriate.

What do you mean, like what? You mean, do I want to hurt my baby? Never! Some women will immediately ask for clarification. Such a response may be indicative of a defensive posture, shielding them from an authentic exploration of their thoughts. If a woman is so frightened by her own thoughts that she is defensive about the question, she may not be able to answer, even with a sensitive clinician. In addition, lack of understanding as to why the question is being asked will likely lead to suspicious or self-protective reactions.

After posing the initial assessment question, a provider might find it helpful to expand the questioning with more specific prompts: *Are you having any thoughts that are scaring you about hurting yourself or your baby? Are you having any troubling thoughts that seem to come out of nowhere over and over again?* This line of questioning is not intended to judge a woman's mothering, even though it can feel that way. It's a critical part of early assessment and lets women know that scary thoughts are common during the postpartum period. By and large, women are relieved to discover that their thoughts are shared by others and are not necessarily a worrisome phenomenon. This early intervention is one of the first ways to peel back the layers of defense that could otherwise obscure the clinical picture. By acknowledging the anxiety associated with uncontrollable scary thoughts, the clinician offers reassurance and immediate relief, thereby reducing the feelings of shame and establishing trust.

When considering aspects of the clinical environment, it is reasonable to presume that the setting is directly related to a woman's readiness (or lack thereof) to disclose. For this reason, efforts to increase awareness of maternal mental health issues have focused not only on educating providers regarding assessment and treatment protocols, but also on empowering the mother to become her own best health advocate.

The bottom line is this: The experience of having scary thoughts means different things to everyone. This includes healthcare providers and the women who are struggling with these thoughts. New mothers will be more inclined to seek help when they can trust that they are being cared for by healthcare providers who understand the implications of the stressors of new motherhood and their impact on the way a woman thinks and feels. It is reasonable that, until women feel safe in this way, they will continue to be wary when these questions are asked. Shame, embarrassment, and fear continue to take center stage for the woman who harbors thoughts that are scaring her. Finding the right place to express this and feel safe is paramount.

There are many instances in which aspects of postpartum distress are missed. Postpartum depression is often a highly agitated depression, presenting with anxiety that can be, for many women, as distressing and debilitating as depressive symptoms. These high levels of distress can lead to widespread misunderstanding and misdiagnosis. Katherine Dalton, a British pioneer in the study of women with postpartum depression, points out that anxiety is the first on her list of complaints from women with postpartum depression. This is followed by insomnia, agitation, and irritability, with symptoms of depression falling into 10th place on the list (Dalton, 1996).

It follows that if current depression scales concentrate on depressive symptoms and fail to identify significant anxiety-related symptoms, it is imperative that healthcare practitioners be skilled at addressing the seriousness and full range of these symptoms as part of their assessment. Screening tools are part of the solution, but the larger issue rests with improving outcomes by enhancing clinical practice and paying specific attention to the matter of anxiety-related scary thoughts.

It has been estimated that 50% of women with postpartum distress have symptoms that remain undetected (Peindl, Wisner, & Hanusa, 2004). A likely explanation is that this results from women's disinclination to disclose and providers' lack of screening knowledge. If healthcare providers do not ask every single postpartum woman if she is having thoughts that are scaring her, they have no way of knowing whether she is experiencing distressing thoughts or not. To presume that she is not, simply because she looks good or says all the right things, will be ineffectual at best and, at worst, disastrous when it prolongs or aggravates the suffering. Thus, even if we envision that perfect scenario when all postpartum women are universally and routinely screened, the issue of asking the right questions remains a high priority.

The first step to increase the likelihood that a woman will confess how she is feeling is to educate providers and consumers alike about the concept of scary thoughts. Knowledge in this area will facilitate appropriate actions and promote faster healing. It would not be fair to expect family practitioners, obstetricians, pediatricians, or midwives (or mothers-in-law, for that matter) to assume the role of a psychiatrist. Nevertheless, these providers see many more postpartum women than do psychiatrists, and it behooves them to have a basic understanding of postpartum distress.

Women are frustrated and are responding with great passion as they share their personal accounts and identify with the stories of others that are splashed across the blogosphere. As social networking has soared, so has the opportunity to utilize this medium to advance public awareness and reduce the isolation of those that are suffering. In the relative anonymity of cyberspace, women find a safe haven where they feel comfortable writing what they might otherwise withhold. Most often, their words are embraced by others, either anonymous or familiar, who convey gratitude for the candid expression to which they can relate. As reliance on the Internet continues to rise, this interchange has enormous psycho-supportive power and has shown to be of great value.

However, as briefly mentioned in the previous chapter, the Internet can also be a precarious place for women with acute anxiety who may by highly suggestible or cling to erroneous claims promoted by unsubstantiated sources. Extreme caution should be exercised regarding the use of the Internet when symptoms or scary thoughts are troublesome and treatment has not yet been initiated. We will examine the use of online support further in Chapter 7.

As stated in the book's preface, in the early stages of our proposal for this book, the publisher had concerns about using our voices to speak to two target audiences simultaneously: consumers and treating clinicians. Our publisher raised a legitimate marketability issue as well as more logistical matters, such as the tone of our writing and readability. How does one write to readers with such divergent agendas? Understandably, harboring a scary thought is a far cry from treating one.

But we believed strongly that both populations would benefit from this information. We presumed that much of what we wrote on behalf of clinical intervention for scary thoughts would be interesting and pertinent to postpartum women experiencing the phenomenon. Women have been asking for this. Some use their voices, some use written words, and some use their deafening stillness and withdrawal. All say the same thing: They want to be heard and understood. And they want to feel better. They search voraciously for information and validation. They are on a mission to help themselves and to help others who suffer in the same way. The solidarity that develops among these women is inspiring, and the camaraderie that fuels their huge undertaking to better educate themselves, their communities, and their healthcare providers is equally impressive.

ROUTINE SCREENING

Even the best-trained providers may not be able to tell if a woman is experiencing symptoms of PPD [postpartum depression] simply by the way she looks or presents in a clinical visit. For this reason, it is critical to routinely screen all postpartum women for PPD. Consider this screening as if you were measuring any other health indicator, such as blood pressure, temperature, or weight. (STEP-PPD: Support and Training to Enhance Primary Care for Postpartum Depression)

It may seem obvious that both consumers and healthcare practitioners should strive for optimal communication in order to maximize clinical care and outcome. Yet, gaps in this area continue to interrupt the continuity of care. One study of family physicians in Washington showed that although the physicians believed postpartum distress was a serious, identifiable, and treatable condition, screening was not standard procedure and the use of screening tools specifically designed for postpartum depression was uncommon (Seehusen, Baldwin, Runkle, & Clark, 2005).

Routine office screenings for common medical conditions that might otherwise go undiagnosed and untreated have been shown to increase recognition and treatment of these conditions (Geogiopoulos, Bryan, Wollan, & Yawn, 2001). Thus far, routine screening for postpartum distress is not common in the United States. Resistance to general screening practices for postpartum distress varies from a general misunderstanding of the nature of this distress to the occupational hazard of implementing psychiatric screening in general practitioner, pediatric, or obstetric settings.

With respect to postpartum depression, studies have shown that screening in the outpatient setting improves the rates of detection and treatment (Geogiopoulos et al., 2001). There are screening tools designed and validated for use with postpartum women, such as the Edinburgh Postnatal Depression Scale (EPDS) (Cox, Holden, & Sagovsky, 1987), Postpartum Checklist (Beck, 1995), and the Postpartum Depression Screening Scale (PDSS) (Beck & Gable, 2000), but none of these specifically targets anxiety symptoms. The EPDS includes three items that pertain to anxiety, but those items are better able to detect postpartum depression than any one anxiety disorder (Kabir, Sheeder, & Kelly, 2008). At the time of this writing, there is no established screening tool for postpartum anxiety, nor is there an established screening tool for scary thoughts.

There is much controversy regarding universal screening for postpartum depression. Recently, the Melanie Blocker-Stokes Postpartum Depression Research and Care Act, also known as the Mother's Act, became a law that mandates funding for research, services, and public education on behalf of women with postpartum depression. Advocates of this law assert that an increase in awareness and services would, in turn, increase identification of symptomatic postpartum women who might otherwise fall through the cracks of the medical system. Opponents of the law claim that there is a risk of false positive outcomes and the potential for widespread overdiagnosis and overmedication.

Regardless of one's personal or professional stance on this law, there are an astounding 2,680,000 to 3,640,000 postpartum women per year with or without a diagnosis of postpartum depression who may experience scary thoughts. It is recommended that healthcare providers attend to this reality responsibly and with compassion, by using the one-question screen for each postpartum woman in their practice: *Are you having any thoughts that are scaring you?* This is a question that should be asked of every single postpartum woman in any and all healthcare contexts.

Relationship With One's Provider

Research shows that primary care providers most often identify postpartum distress (41.3%), followed by obstetricians (30.7%), and mental health providers (13.0%) (Dietz et al., 2007). Because a woman's history of depression and anxiety is a significant risk factor for postpartum distress (Wisner, Chambers, & Sit, 2006), all providers should be diligent about gathering relevant history. The same principle applies to current information that might contribute to the manner in which a woman is currently feeling or may feel during the postpartum period (e.g., marital issues, environmental stressors, baby-related pressures, job stress). Understandably, each provider has his or her area of expertise and perspective. However, with increased awareness and education, there is great potential for each medical discipline to find its own way past resistance and to the heart of a postpartum woman.

Remember the paradox of this resistance: Postpartum women yearn to be heard and understood, yet are often paralyzed by their fears. Taking the risk of trusting a healthcare provider who may not respond with the appropriate empathy and action poses a greater threat than some women are willing to take. Therefore, when treating postpartum women, it would be prudent for providers to consider the stigma and surrounding issues (e.g., her reluctance to share how she is feeling) and keep in mind that women will be more likely to disclose when the process is initiated with careful attention to the nature of this resistance.

There are two primary venues for routine depression screening for postpartum women: the mother's postpartum office visits (i.e., obstetrician, family practice physicians, nurse-midwives) and the infant's well-child visits (i.e., pediatricians, family practice physician) (Gjerdingen & Yawn, 2007). In the following sections, we discuss potential screening practices as we consider the influence of some specific healthcare providers on a postpartum woman and her willingness to discuss how she is feeling.

The Pediatrician

In a national survey, 57% of pediatricians reported that they believed they were responsible for identifying postpartum depression, but only 32% expressed confidence in their ability to diagnose it (Olson et al., 2002). One of the primary reasons pediatricians have been the focus of increased attention with respect to postpartum distress screening is the awareness that they may be the only healthcare practitioner whom mothers see on a regular basis (Chaudron, 2003). Linda Chaudron, a pediatrician who has written extensively on bringing the practice of screening for postpartum depression into pediatric offices, has broken new ground by attempting to bridge the two specialties of pediatrics and psychiatry. She deems that pediatricians play a central role in coordinating with other medical providers regarding screening practices.

Although Chaudron suggests that this screening falls within the scope of pediatric practice, it is not without its flaws. Perhaps the biggest obstacle is the notion that the pediatrician is the baby's doctor, not the mother's. This alone leads to a number of potential distractions from both perspectives; the primary one is a mother's reluctance to present herself as anything less than a healthy mother. Additionally, because pediatricians do not provide adult care, one could argue that they are not sufficiently prepared to manage adult mental health issues and referrals.

Leslie, a first-time mother of 5-month-old twins, suppressed her secret wish that she had only given birth to one baby. After 4 years of infertility treatments along with her lifelong desire to have a baby, she could hardly bear her intermittent fantasy that she had given birth to only one baby. She was exhausted and overwhelmed, and she generally felt incapable of managing the needs of two babies simultaneously. She was especially troubled when she singled out one of the twins, the one who was more consolable and easier for her to handle, as her preferred baby.

Leslie believed it would be better if she weren't their mother: *Perhaps I could just leave, and no one would notice.* Bringing her babies for their check-up was always agitating for her. The office visits gave rise to her fear that the doctor would see that she didn't like being a mother. She feared he would detect her ever present thoughts of wishing away one of the babies. Imagine how unnerving it would be for her to hear the babies' doctor ask: *Are you having any thoughts that are scaring you?*

As with screening for any condition, the tool or the process is only as effective as the skills of the screener, the reliability of the responses, and the appropriateness of follow-through. Anyone can read a series of questions placed in front of her, hand out a 10-item questionnaire to a patient, or, as with Leslie, simply ask a question in a forthright manner. In order to increase the probability that responses will be truthful, pediatricians need to consider the connection they have with that patient. And, reciprocally, the woman needs to consider her relationship with her baby's doctor before she responds.

Ann Heneghan, a pediatrician in Cleveland, found that mothers were particularly responsive to pediatricians whose style of communication suggested that they cared for the mother's well-being (Heneghan, Mercer, & DeLeone, 2004). Using quotes directly from women who had sought support at her focus groups (Heneghan et al., 2004, p. 464), she compiled a useful list of communication do's and don'ts for pediatricians. These suggestions were as follows:

Do ...
    "Respect my opinions."
    "Take time to listen."
    "Anticipate my concerns."
    "Talk to my child/care about my child."
    "Ask me the right questions."
    "Ask; I would answer."
Don't ...
    "Judge me."
    "Cut me short."
    "Talk down to me."

In short, women in this study were in agreement that pediatricians who conveyed that they cared, through sensitive screening, were more likely to elicit honest responses to their questions than those who did not. When a pediatrician fails to recognize the value of this role, a mother's anxiety can remain undetected, and she is left to continue parenting her baby with high levels of anxiety and potential impairment. Ultimately, of course, this affects the child's well-being and creates the inevitable loop back to the pediatrician's target patient. The 2-, 6-, and 12-month well-baby appointments with pediatricians or family physicians have been noted as reasonable opportunities to use a brief screening tool for postpartum anxiety and depression (Clay & Seehusen, 2004).

The Obstetrician or Midwife

Though some practices have combined obstetric and midwifery services, many women have strong feelings about their decision to use one over the other. In this book, we use the word obstetrician to include both. As pointed out in Chapter 5, the self-report questionnaire at The Postpartum Stress Center revealed that the overwhelming majority of clients distinguished the obstetrician as the healthcare provider to whom they were most likely to disclose any of their distressing thoughts. Women tended to be in agreement that the obstetrician–patient dyad is an intimate and ongoing (especially throughout pregnancy) professional relationship that provides a preestablished comfort zone—so much so, that a surprising number of women reported having no doctor other than their obstetrician.

In contrast to the pediatrician, the obstetrician may pose less of a perceived threat to the postpartum woman because he or she is not the baby's doctor and is a direct link to the pregnancy and postpartum experience. Moreover, many women tell us they are not interested in seeing a psychiatrist at this time and prefer the convenience and comfort of their established relationship with their obstetrician. It is important to acknowledge that although some say they'd rather not see a "shrink" if they don't have to, just as many women are relieved to see a medical doctor who specializes in the treatment of emotional illness. It does seem to be the case, however, that in this time of managed healthcare systems and unclear pathways to symptom relief, the obstetrician is often seen by postpartum women as the gatekeeper for medical services.

Another way that an obstetrician can help is to recognize when a woman is at an increased risk for anxiety or depression during pregnancy or even before becoming pregnant. This awareness will help a woman at risk identify issues and seek treatment at an earlier point than she might have otherwise done.

One notable obstacle is that the obstetrician and the woman herself may believe that the doctor's job is complete after the baby is born; this notion would inhibit the mother from reaching out for help (Stone, 2008). These unclear boundaries are largely responsible for the likelihood that the needs of postpartum women will fall between the cracks of the medical system. In general, postpartum follow-up care after childbirth consists of one office visit during the 6 weeks after birth. These visits primarily focus on postdelivery recovery, contraception, and general well-being.

Although not all obstetricians have incorporated a systematic investigation of the woman's postpartum emotional adjustment, most are becoming aware that their patients appreciate attention to this aspect of their recovery after childbirth. At this time, there are conflicting recommendations for the timing intervals for screening for postpartum distress in obstetrical practices. However, in light of a recent statement by the American College of Obstetricians and Gynecologists that postpartum depression would be a top priority within the new presidential initiative (American Congress of Obstetricians and Gynecologists, 2009), we suspect that formal guidelines are forthcoming.

The Family Physician

Although studies have found that the more than 80% of mothers indicated being comfortable with the idea of being screened for postpartum depression (Gemmill, Leigh, Ericksen, & Milgrom, 2006), the rate of current screening in primary care settings is below 50% (Seehusen et al., 2005). We have seen that, despite the fact that family physicians perceive postpartum distress as serious, identifiable, and treatable, their use of screening tools designed for postpartum depression is uncommon, and the use of screening tools for anxiety is virtually nonexistent.

However, it is an important area to explore because it is undisputed that postpartum issues impact the entire family. When distress sets in during the postpartum period, fathers are prone to depression, maternal-infant relationships are affected, older children are vulnerable to behavioral problems, and marriages are stressed (Areias, Kumar, Barros, & Figueiredo, 1996). Family physicians are trained to treat the individual as a whole person within the family context. It's a philosophy of practice that is fundamentally suited for postpartum attentiveness and should lend itself to routine screening practices. Postpartum women who are comfortable with their family doctor should consider this relationship and be open to the possibility that this avenue may provide access to symptom relief. If a referral to a mental health specialist is indicated, the family physician can treat in the interim, particularly if there is a wait time to see the specialist.

The Mental Health Provider

Many therapists who may regularly treat individuals, couples, or families may not necessarily be alert to the impact that recent childbirth may have had on the client. Unless therapists are trained or have a special interest in the perinatal (time period before and after birth) population, they might easily miss a prenatal or postpartum diagnosis that could significantly impact the individual and her family. We are hopeful that current attention to these common complications following childbirth will enlighten clinicians who might not have otherwise considered this factor in their assessments.

Screening for postpartum anxiety and depression should be a top priority for clinicians who are treating individuals or couples who have had a baby within the past year. If a couple is being treated, it is recommended that both mother and father be screened because the emergence of significant postpartum distress is possible for both. Screening for postpartum distress should be carried out at the first visit and then repeated at subsequent visits in order to monitor progress.

Mental health specialists are in an optimal position to provide a safe and comfortable outlet for women to reveal how they are feeling. Without a doubt, this is part of the reason that practices that specialize in women's healthcare or specifically in the treatment of postpartum depression are certain to get a higher degree of disclosure. At The Postpartum Stress Center, there is essentially no discrepancy between what women indicate on the detailed screening tools in the waiting room and what they reveal in their first session. In other words, if they check off that they are experiencing scary thoughts about themselves or their babies on the form, they seem to be prepared to open up in session about these specific thoughts. Women say they are initially both relieved and startled to see so many of their own scary thoughts and feelings already in black and white, but that, ultimately, this is validating for them. They have found a safe place.

IT'S A MATTER OF STYLE

If creating a safe environment is the key to augmenting the truthful expression of symptoms or experiences, it is not enough for providers simply to agree to incorporate screening tools into their practices. Providers must take a close look at what they are asking, how they are asking it, and, quite frankly, *why* they are asking and what they plan to do about the responses they might get. Pediatricians, perhaps above all, must be mindful of the manner in which these questions are asked and the manner in which they may be perceived by a nervous woman who is desperately trying to present herself as a good mother.

No one would argue that healthcare providers feel constrained by time limits and insufficient training with regard to postpartum screening. There is a legitimate concern that there is not enough time to counsel adequately and take a thorough history. But because postpartum anxiety disorders and depression remain highly underreported and underdiagnosed (Mancini, Carlson, & Albers, 2007), it becomes necessary to find ways to break through the barriers and augment awareness, training, and screening skill. Despite the compelling and genuine barriers to assessing for scary thoughts, opportunities for appropriate screening *do* exist and need to be executed. The obvious positive outcome is validation and symptom relief; the less obvious but more critical consideration is the impact of a woman's continued distress on her ability to parent and to engage in her marriage.

The vast barriers and the potential value to screening for scary thoughts can be condensed into this concept: Whether or not a woman has been diagnosed with postpartum distress, the likelihood that she is experiencing thoughts that are scaring her is extremely high. All healthcare providers who have contact with postpartum women should feel obliged to address this issue as part of their standard care. Regardless of whether or not a woman is having any thoughts that are scaring her, asking this question in a sensitive and compassionate manner creates a connection between provider and patient that will facilitate effective communication and provide an invaluable foundation of trust for future interventions.

Madeleine, a new mother with postpartum depression, came to The Postpartum Stress Center for support after visiting two previous clinicians who had failed to provide the support she needed. It was hard for Madeleine to find the strength to hunt for qualified clinicians when she felt so depleted. Regrettably, her experience demonstrates the way in which the lack of professional sensitivity can hamper an assessment and evaluation. She described her first visit with a psychiatrist:

> I went to this doctor because a friend of mine had referred her and told me she had experience with postpartum depression. That's hard to believe. First, she asked me a couple of questions about my baby and how I felt about him, you know, like if I was going to hurt him or abandon him or something. Then she looked up from her note-taking frenzy, looked me in the eyes with her furrowed brow, and asked sternly, "You're not thinking about killing yourself, are you?"

Presumably, readers of this book will also be appalled and understand the concept being emphasized here. Asking the question—even the right question—is not necessarily sufficient. How it is asked and the motivation for asking it are equally relevant. A quick Internet search with the words postpartum depression screening tools will lead to descriptions of the various available instruments and numerous testimonies to the ease with which the screening tools can be administered. Phrases like "user friendly," "10 item," "easy to score," "can be completed in approximately 5 minutes," and so on are used to make the screening process more efficient and attractive to physicians who have no time to spare.

But, as we've seen, having that piece of paper is only a fraction of the solution. The success of this entire picture encompasses more of a mindset as opposed merely to utilizing a tool. Healthcare providers need to understand what is at stake and acquire the skills that will enable them to be effective. The list of potential professional contacts who should be alert to the potential for scary thoughts is extensive: obstetricians, pediatricians, physician assistants, midwives, family practice physicians, nurse practitioners, public health nurses, home visitors, lactation consultants, childbirth educators, individual and family psychotherapists, psychiatrists, hospital maternity or neonatal intensive care nurses, nutritionists, maternity clinic staff, and emergency room staff. Even in the absence of an institution's formal screening protocol, practitioners should be conscientious concerning symptoms or experiences that might otherwise be disregarded.

Certain statements and questions and specific words can either deter the admission of scary thoughts or usher a woman into a secure space, thereby increasing the likelihood of disclosure. Therefore, it is incumbent upon healthcare professionals to utilize compassionate and effective assessment techniques. Even when mothers disclose they are having scary thoughts, they often do not disclose all of them or those that are particularly disturbing. Although postpartum women tend not to mention thoughts of killing their babies to healthcare providers, when their thoughts are suicidal in nature, they are more likely to reach out and disclose in order to get the help they need (Barr & Beck, 2008; Meyer & Spinelli, 2003). Thus, when suicidal thoughts are disclosed, healthcare providers should probe further for the possibility that there may be scary thoughts that have not yet been revealed, such as thoughts of harm coming to the infant.

Regardless of any forthright guidance, healthcare providers may remain uncertain as to the specific manner in which they should bring up this sensitive subject. An effective protocol involves five variables. Keep in mind that the first three refer to the *preparation* and the last two refer to the response after the one-question screen: *Are you having any thoughts that are scaring you?* Although the order of these items may appear insignificant at first glance, if the question is asked without adequate preparation, the woman is likely to shut down. If this happens, access to her expression of distress may be irretrievable:

- **Speaking tone.** The tone should be one of compassion. It should convey empathy but not sorrow, excessive worry, or pity. It should be warm, but unemotional. Tones that are either too cold or too sympathetic can be perceived as offensive. An objective but caring manner will impart a sense of control that will be extremely comforting to an anxious woman.
- **Spoken statement of professional's ability to ensure her well-being.** *It is routine for our office to ask questions about a mother's emotional health after she has a baby.* A statement of this nature will confirm that the mother is in good hands and that she is not the first person who has ever expressed concern about the way she is feeling.
- **Spoken statement of validation.** Validation of the occurrence of scary thoughts is the most important unwritten rule. *It is common for new mothers to experience thoughts that are scary to them. Sometimes it's hard to talk about these thoughts.* These statements convey that the provider to some extent expects this level of distress and also understands the internal struggle. This provides a welcome reprieve, whether or not a woman decides to disclose at that time.

- **Direct question of experience (one-question screen).** *Are you having any thoughts that are scaring you?* This may require explanation or further clarification of what is being asked, particularly for women who are not having this experience. Women who are experiencing this will know exactly what the question means.
- **Repeat validation.** Whether or not a woman discloses at this point, the provider should reiterate the fact that this is common. It is not an indication that anything terrible is going on; rather, it is often associated with the high demands and anxiety present with motherhood.

FOLLOWING UP

It is helpful for the healthcare provider always to leave the door open by providing options in the event that the woman needs additional attention. These can be simple references, such as: *Be sure to call the office if you need anything; don't hesitate to let me know if you are worried about the way you are feeling; if anything changes or concerns you before our next appointment, let me know.* Statements such as these will be reassuring and demonstrate the high level of care that is available to the woman.

Postpartum anxiety and depression are serious conditions that are currently receiving long overdue attention, and various healthcare providers are working diligently to make a difference. Healthcare providers need to augment their screening practices, clinical interviews, and referral practices in order to maximize access to effective treatment and follow-up care. In addition, a comprehensive mental health evaluation should always follow screening that is positive or if a problem is suspected.

Take-Home Point for Mothers. If you are having scary thoughts, make sure you are in the right place. Do not presume healthcare providers know how bad you are feeling. If they fail to ask you directly, let them know how they can best help you. If you do not feel comfortable enough to do this, bring a support person with you or consider that you might need to find another provider who can better meet your needs.

Clinician Note. A universal, one-question screen is *Are you having thoughts that are scaring you?* Ask this question of every pregnant and postpartum woman in your practice. If her response is *no*, continue to ask it again each time you see her. She may not be ready to tell you yet. Because almost all postpartum women experience scary thoughts from time to time, it is safe to presume that most of your postpartum clients or patients are having some. Initiate this important dialogue with kindness and directness and as part of a thorough assessment.

Section III

Breaking the Cycle of Scary Thoughts

7

Things You Can Do to Feel Better

I swear I was possessed. It was like one part of my brain was off on its own with stabbing thoughts that didn't make sense to the other side of my brain. I felt like a stranger in my own body, almost like I was there and not there at the same time. It was weird. I told no one how I was feeling. Absolutely no one. I believed if I told anyone how I was feeling they would surely think I had lost my mind. Everything looked good on the outside so I just pretended everything was fine. I mean, no one could tell there was so much chaos in my head. But the thoughts would pierce through my brain when I least expected it, usually when I was bathing the baby. Bath time took only as long as I could hold my breath and get it over with. I didn't know what else to do.

Jen, 5 months postpartum

Dealing with scary thoughts is not just a matter of willpower, as some claim. Although willpower may indeed be part of the solution, we've seen throughout this book that it is more complicated than simply wishing thoughts away. We've all heard the truism that if we think positively, we'll feel better. Sounds good, doesn't it? Research has shown that one of the most significant attributions for recovery from anxiety or depression seems to be the individual's belief in her ability to take control and be successful (Kinnier, Hofsess, Pongratz, & Lambert, 2009). In other words, if someone believes she will be successful, she is more likely to succeed.

For our purposes here, even though some of the suggestions may feel counterintuitive at first, it will be helpful for you to believe that some of what you read in this chapter will help you feel better. Though we realize it is much easier said than done, great personal power can come from shifting the focus of your energy from fear (negative) to acceptance (positive). For mild to moderate degrees of distress, women report that they feel more in control of their lives when they take responsibility for how they are feeling and identify the specific actions they can take to feel better.

In Chapter 5, we discussed the barriers to disclosure, or those things that get in the way of women speaking up about how they are feeling—the critical voice, the sentencing factor, the depression factor, the ambiguity factor, the propaganda factor, the community factor, and the what-if factor. All of these impediments combine to create a setting that discourages women from admitting they are having scary thoughts. Due to the high degree of distress you may be experiencing with your scary thoughts, our attention now turns to some specific self-help strategies you can rely on to ease the impact of your anxiety, depression, and scary thoughts. As you read, keep these six principles in mind:

- Denying the feelings and thoughts will not make them go away.
- Panicking will make them worse.
- Resistance creates persistence.
- Distraction will help for a while.
- Enhancing awareness might feel counterintuitive, but it is meaningful.
- Acceptance is hard but essential.

WHAT *WON'T* HELP: COUNTERPRODUCTIVE REACTIONS

Most women respond to the distress of scary thoughts with mechanisms that are called upon to protect them from emotional pain. Some might refuse to believe the thoughts are there (denial). Others might try desperately to make the thoughts go away (thought suppression). Another common response is to react with sudden, intense fear that interferes with the ability to function (panic). Although these three responses are quite common and understandable, they will not help you feel better, and they can even make you feel worse.

Denial

One of the first responses reported by postpartum women with scary thoughts is denial. *Maybe if I just pretend it isn't happening, it will go away.*

Denial serves to protect people emotionally. In some instances, it can be temporarily adaptive, such as when someone is forced to deal with the reality of unbearable news. Likewise, this common psychological defense seems to soften the blow of scary thoughts. However, when someone refuses to or simply cannot accept the certainty of a situation over time, denial is viewed as maladaptive. Because scary thoughts are so often accompanied by feelings of shame and the belief that one is damaged in some way, they often are wished away with fierce determination. Many women who are having scary thoughts believe it would feel better to pretend they weren't there. Sometimes this is evident from the initial phone call to the clinician:

"Are you having any thoughts that are scaring you?"

"No."

"Is there anything else you would like me to know before we set up the appointment?"

"Not really."

"Then let me take a look and find a time for you to come in as soon as possible so that you can start to feel better."

"Okay … um … uh … I … I'm not having thoughts of hurting my baby or anything. My doctor asked me that and I'm not having thoughts like that."

"Okay. Are you having any other thoughts that might be worrying you? It might feel better if you tell me now before we meet. Perhaps I can reassure you, so you don't have to worry so much in the meantime."

"No. Everything's fine. I'm just crying all the time. I'll be okay until our appointment."

Women would rather not admit that they are having scary thoughts, at least not at first. The denial we are talking about here is slightly different from the unconscious, ego-protective defense mechanism taught in Psychology 101. Here, the denial is more of a conscious or deliberate attempt to shield one from the reality that feels so unacceptable. The distorted belief is that *if I don't put words to it, it isn't really happening.*

The benefit that comes from denial is a short-term reprieve. Essentially, what it does is grant some time to adjust. After all, having a scary thought, however fleeting or purposeless, can be unsettling. The refusal to acknowledge it becomes a stumbling block in the long run because it prevents one from taking action that could help alleviate one's stress. In this way, denial is self-sabotaging by directly interfering with the management of scary thoughts, as well as postponing relief from them.

Thought Suppression

We've seen that denial can surface as an immediate reaction to uncomfortable states of anxiety; it also requires a substantial investment of energy. Because of this, other defenses may be called upon. *Thought suppression* is the deliberate act of trying to force the unwanted information out of your awareness.

Remember the old brain teaser: "For the next 2 minutes, think about anything you want, but you cannot think about pink elephants. Think about whatever you want, but you must not think about pink elephants!" Of course, everyone reports seeing one or more big pink elephants in the mind's eye immediately after being told to suppress that image.

Over 20 years ago, a study was carried out to test the prediction that a person's attempt to suppress thoughts can result in preoccupation with that thought—a phenomenon the researchers referred to as a *rebound effect* (Wegner, Schneider, Carter, & White, 1987). In this experiment, participants were asked to speak spontaneously for 5 minutes straight, talking about anything and everything. Next, they were again asked to verbalize everything that came to mind, but this time they were told not to think about a white bear. They were instructed to ring a bell each time they said or thought "white bear." Interestingly, when compared to a group that was told to think about white bears, the group that was asked to suppress white bear thoughts had significantly *more* thoughts on this topic.

The researchers concluded that attempts at thought suppression had a paradoxical effect, suggesting that suppression might produce the very thought it is intended to stifle. Subsequent research has supported this notion and confirms repeated failure by people to suppress unwanted thoughts (Wenzlaff & Wegner, 2000). In other words, thought suppression just does not work.

This work has strong implications with regard to thought control as a self-help strategy for postpartum women with scary thoughts. Most postpartum women will admit that their initial instinct is to suppress the thought; quite simply, they want to make the bad thought go away by trying not to think about it. The notion that it is unhealthy and even dangerous to stifle emotions and bottle them up inside is not a new one. But the message here is an important one: The instinctive response to control a scary thought by holding it in or concealing it typically backfires and makes things feel worse. Persistence creates resistance; the more you try to push thoughts out, the bigger they get.

This paradox was described in *Therapy and the Postpartum Woman* (Kleiman, 2008) using the metaphor of a filled water balloon. Imagine trying to control a wobbly water balloon resting precariously in the palm of one's hand. Your instinct is to grab it as it rolls from side to side. But in doing so, you find that the overstuffed balloon either pops out of your gripping fingers and onto the floor, or it bursts right within your grasp into a sopping mess. Either way, control has been lost. The only way to gain control over an unsteady water balloon is to release your fingers, slowly open your hand, and let go of the tight grip. This exercise demonstrates the paradox of control. Letting go when you are overwhelmed and frightened is difficult and can feel counterproductive, but it works. We say more about letting go at the end of this chapter.

Panic

Negative self-talk can trigger or aggravate a state of acute anxiety. Karen refers to this as an "uh-oh" response: *Oh no, I'm having that thought again. Uh-oh, here it comes again. Oh my God, now I won't be able to do what I need to do. Oh what if I get sick again like the last time? I can't do anything; oh no, I can't breathe. I really cannot breathe.* This snapshot of a paralyzing moment in time demonstrates the power of negative thinking and the manner in which it can escalate from one short exclamation into a blast of memories or associations. If one is experiencing panic, recognizing the thoughts that precipitate this barrage of emotion is an important step toward relief. In the next chapter, we will examine some specific strategies to help restructure negative thinking into more productive patterns.

Panic and negative thoughts have a reciprocal relationship; that is, one contributes to the other. Knowing this can promote both awareness and management of the scary thoughts. If a postpartum woman is in treatment for anxiety or depression, she will notice that as her anxiety is successfully managed, her scary thoughts will likewise decrease in degree and/or severity. This is because, as stated previously, it is not the content of the scary thought that is noteworthy; rather, it is the level of distress it causes. Thus, even though a woman may be preoccupied with the content (*Why would I have a picture in my head of my baby lying in a coffin on the beach?*), trained clinicians will focus their intervention away from the specific content and toward treatment of the anxiety.

Panic has the innate capacity to undo lots of hard work. Jen felt for sure that she was driving herself crazy. She knew she didn't have any good reason to worry so much.

> "Does anyone?" she would ask. "I mean, yes, I know some people have real reason to worry, God knows. So that makes me feel guilty, of course. But don't most people who worry a lot worry for no good reason?"
>
> "What do you mean, 'no good reason'?" Karen asked.
>
> "I mean my baby is healthy. My husband is awesome. I have everything I've ever wanted. I should feel great, but I don't. I worry about everything. And nothing. And then, BAM!! Just when I think my brain is coasting along for a slow ride, I smack into some nasty insane thought about some God-awful thing happening to my baby or my husband. Slam! Right out of nowhere."
>
> "That's a terrible feeling, especially when you're not expecting it. What do you do when that happens?"
>
> "Oh my God, I freak. I can't breathe, and I start to sweat. My whole body shakes like I have a chill or something."
>
> "Do you know what you're thinking when you are feeling that way?"
>
> "Yeah. I'm thinking, '*Shit,* I can't believe this is happening again!!' "

Jen was a 33-year-old mother of two, with the youngest only a few weeks old. Unlike her sister, who experienced significant anxiety growing up, Jen was unfamiliar with this agitated state and even seemed to dodge it after her first child was born. But with her second baby, she was overcome with anxiety from the start. Each day brought unfamiliar waves of uneasiness that made her wonder if something really awful was happening to her. During those times when she felt less anxiety, she would feel closer to her wish that all of her scary thoughts and feelings would magically disappear. Then, BAM (as she described it)—an unwanted thought would strike like an electrical jolt, setting aflame every worry she could possibly imagine. The worst, of course, was worry about harm coming to her baby.

Jen's resistance to her anxious thoughts created the perfect setting for panic, which then found its way right to the heart of her vulnerability—harm coming to her baby. Here's an oversimplification of what was happening: When a woman experiences a scary thought, she can go down one of two roads. She can say or think, *Okay, I know what this is. I understand this is an irrational thought and has nothing to do with what is really going to happen or not happen. I can try to distract myself. Maybe I'll call my friend.* On the other hand, she can say and/or think, *Oh my God, why is this happening again?! I thought I was okay. I thought this wasn't going to happen again. Maybe I really am going crazy. What do I do?!* Jen's "uh-oh" response is an example of this second response. That road is more likely to increase feelings of helplessness, loss of control, and panic.

The core principle behind the first response is learning to refocus and label scary thoughts as unwanted and, more importantly, unthreatening. This takes practice and is typically not intuitive. The knee-jerk reaction for most postpartum women, particularly those with a predisposition to anxiety, will be to charge down the second road. It seems automatic, sometimes, to do what's familiar, even if it accentuates the mental stress.

Choosing the first road requires a deliberate decision to respond differently by modifying the usual response with an unfamiliar, more practical one in order to achieve a better outcome. It's easy to imagine in theory. *All you have to do is respond differently, and you won't panic as much!* Sure. Easier said than done. Nevertheless, understanding that you *do* have power over how you feel is an enormous victory. Putting it into practice and believing in your capacity to follow through is the next step.

WHAT *WILL* HELP: SELF-HELP STRATEGIES AND NONPROFESSIONAL INTERVENTIONS

We've seen that denial, thought suppression, and panic not only don't work, but also will frequently intensify the distress. Though it's easy to understand how these responses would be knee-jerk reactions to an insufferable state—*This can't be happening. Oh my God! Stop it, make it go away*—learning how to dial down those reactive states and activate constructive responses is a priority at this time. If reactions such as those don't help, what does?

Self-help strategies and nonprofessional treatment options include those in which postpartum women seek help on their own or along with their peers and do not involve a healthcare professional to lead or guide. Women pursue these options for a variety of reasons, including time and scheduling limitations, financial restrictions, maintaining a sense of control, and gaining a feeling of empowerment. Additionally, much less stigma is associated with self-help and peer group interventions than with professional treatment. We will discuss professional treatment options in great length in Chapter 9.

Distraction

Although it may strike you as psychologically unsound, distraction has been shown to be an effective intervention and has been associated with the reduction of distressed mood (Broderick, 2005). At first glance, it may seem to contradict the concept of learning to accept the presence of scary thoughts; however, distraction has been shown to interrupt the loop of negative thinking temporarily. This is not the same thing as avoidance or denial. Rather, it is a way to remain *in* the stressful situation by coping with it. Results from one study suggest that when thoughts were particularly repugnant, people were able to reduce their level of distress significantly by deliberately engaging in distraction or intentionally focusing on a different thought (Najmi, Riemann, & Wegner, 2009). These studies lend credence to the use of distraction as a valid psychological intervention worth exploring further.

Everyone is familiar with the power of distraction. Think about how many mothers successfully maneuver their toddler away from that candy store by bringing attention to something else that excites the child. Or consider the brilliant innovation of installing a DVD player at eye level for patients sitting in the dentist chair!

If you are terrified of your scary thoughts, can you really distract yourself from this uncomfortable mental state? Yes. When you feel fear taking hold, do something that feels manageable. When you engage in work or activity that feels manageable in the present, you minimize your involvement with anxiety-generating thoughts and images and keep the mind actively focused. Your body, in response, is able to settle down a bit, allowing you to feel more in control.

The following list contains just a few examples. Clearly, the categories are arbitrary and overlap. We merely separated them to make the point that people attribute varying degrees of meaning to different activities:

It can be pleasing:
- Flipping through a magazine
- Listening to music
- Watching TV
- Making a phone call to a friend

It can be absorbing:
- Engaging in work-related projects
- Planting in the garden
- Helping a neighbor
- Making a scrapbook with baby pictures
- Playing computer games
- Reading a novel by a favorite author

It can be detail-oriented:
- Doing puzzles or playing games
- Counting the tiles in the ceiling
- Writing
- Organizing
- Counting backward by threes from 100

It can be physical/bodily:
- Snapping a rubber band on wrist
- Visualizing and repeating the word STOP
- Splashing ice cold water on the face
- Gently slapping the cheek
- Talking or reading aloud

It can be energizing:
- Exercising
- Taking a brisk walk in the sunshine
- Dancing

These distraction techniques work to take the mind away temporarily from the worrisome thought and redirect it to something that feels different. This is based on the principle that your brain can perform a limited amount of functions at one time. By keeping your brain busy as much as you can, you are less able to accommodate the anxiety. This is not as easy as it might sound. Keeping your brain busy requires a dedicated effort; it will not be enough to turn on the television and let your brain wander. Before you know it, your thoughts will meander right back to the object of your obsession. It requires a deliberate desire to absorb yourself in an activity.

Count, read, paint, design, clean. Teach your brain how good it can feel to focus on something other than your scary thought. Your thinking is getting in your way right now. Give yourself permission to play and not to think.

In our clinical practices, many women report that they are able to attain a higher degree of comfort when combining distraction techniques with self-soothing behaviors. Self-soothing involves incorporating one or more of your senses (i.e., sight, hearing, smell, taste, touch); such efforts can bring focus to an anxious mind. For instance, you can look at a beautiful scene in nature or a picture of something that feels good to you. Listen to the birds singing. Smell the flowers, or the air outside, or the cookies baking. Enjoy your favorite food or treat yourself to something you can savor for the first time. Cuddle with someone you love. Pet your dog or cat or snuggle up with your favorite old stuffed animal. All of these self-soothing techniques can tame the wild thoughts, if only briefly. The underlying principle is simply that a worried state and a relaxed state are incompatible. That is, it is hard for your brain to worry and truly engage in a pleasurable activity at the same time.

We have mentioned that some worriers hold strong convictions regarding the positive value of their worrying. For these women, worry serves as a sort of insurance investment. *The more I worry about something happening, the more I protect myself and those I love from it actually happening.* When such beliefs are deeply ingrained, a woman might be far less motivated to distract herself. Nonetheless, we strongly encourage you to try using distraction techniques as a means of finding some relief.

Breathing, Relaxation, and Mindfulness

Anxiety is more than just a feeling. When the mind is anxious, the rest of the body kicks into high gear. The heart starts pounding, breathing becomes rapid and shallow, muscles tighten, and one can feel dizzy or disoriented. In addition to the emotional strain and impact on negative thought processes, anxiety can deplete energy reserves and cause a host of physical, emotional, and cognitive problems, such as restlessness, irritability, fatigue, aching, sleep problems, and difficulty concentrating.

It follows, then, that when a woman is a chronic worrier, her body exists in a fixed state of tension. It is for this reason that so many antianxiety strategies emphasize relaxation techniques: They reverse these reactions. In a relaxed state, the heart rate slows down, breathing becomes more controlled and slower, muscles loosen, and blood pressure stabilizes. Research bears out that relaxation exercises work by calming the body and quieting the mind. Learning to breathe in a controlled manner and to refine the relaxation response takes time and practice, but it can pay off in both the short and long run (Davis, Eshelman, & McKay, 2000).

In this section, we briefly describe some common breathing and relaxation strategies. There are varying guidelines depending on the source and the philosophy to which one subscribes. In general, it is recommended that you wear comfortable clothing, find a quiet spot, and set aside anywhere from 10 to 20 minutes a day for these exercises. Some women claim they are too wired or too busy to relax or that these techniques do not work for them. If your base emotional state or your current level of anxiety is high, you might feel discouraged before even attempting these. Still, we would urge you to try one of these methods and see if, with continued practice, they can help you feel better. In fact, taking 10–20 minutes to practice self-care, such as breathing, relaxation, or mindfulness, can make you more productive and centered despite the fact that you took time away from your schedule.

For a portion of women, this exercise feels threatening or impossible. Often, the more anxious you are, the more challenging it can be to practice these exercises, and it's possible to experience emotional discomfort from the feelings evoked by them. If you start the exercise and feel too vulnerable or your anxiety increases, simply stop.

Controlled Breathing

Most people have trouble breathing when they are anxious. Breathing can become rapid and shallow, which can lead to hyperventilation in some cases. Learning to breathe in a controlled manner can help restore a feeling of composure. This type of rhythmic breathing comes from your diaphragm around your abdomen, not your chest, and is sometimes called "belly breathing" (Kabat-Zinn, 1990). Place one hand on your chest and the other on your belly. Inhale as you take a deep breath from your abdomen. As you inhale, you should feel your belly expand. The hand on your chest should not move. After a brief pause, slowly exhale, keeping your focus on your breathing. Your belly should go back down as you exhale. Your complete attention should remain on each breath. It is recommended that you make time to do this for 15 minutes each day, whether or not you feel like it. With regular practice, your breathing can be used as a tool to help combat anxiety.

There is a good reason why controlled breathing works: Anxiety is associated with a sense of uncontrollability and unpredictability, and when your breathing becomes heightened by anxiety, it makes these perceptions that much stronger. Gaining control over your breathing helps to have predictability over one important part of the physiology of anxiety, and the perception of controllability and predictability then extends to other parts of your life. Be sure not to breathe too deeply or too quickly because taking in too much air can disrupt the balance between oxygen and carbon dioxide; this can make your breathing seem more out of control, rather than less.

Progressive Muscle Relaxation

This technique usually begins with controlled breathing and involves tensing and releasing different muscle groups in your body. Take several controlled breaths, as instructed before. Start with your feet and gradually move upward, tensing and then relaxing muscles throughout your body until you finish with muscles in your neck and face. When you tighten each muscle, take note of how the tension feels. Hold this position for 5–10 seconds and quickly release the tension. Stay relaxed for 20–30 seconds. Repeat with each muscle group throughout your body.

Mindfulness Meditation

Meditation has been practiced for centuries and offers great relief for anxious states. It has been claimed that regular mindfulness practice may improve mood and anxiety symptoms by reducing the inclination to react to negative states with ruminative thought or maladaptive behavior (Toneatto & Nguyen 2007). Kabat-Zinn defines mindfulness as the "awareness that emerges through paying attention on purpose, in the present moment, and nonjudgmentally to the unfolding of experience moment by moment" (Kabat-Zinn, 2003, p. 45). In other words, mindfulness requires that you focus your attention on the present moment and reject the temptation to critique the past or worry about the future. Do not judge the moment as good or as bad. It just *is,* and each moment is different from and independent of the previous or future moment.

Here is but one of many mindfulness exercises. Sit comfortably with your eyes closed, with your back upright. Relax and take note of your bodily sensations and the sounds around you. Notice them without judgment. Let your mind settle into the rhythm of breathing as noted before. When it wanders, gently redirect your attention to your breathing. Being aware of your breathing means you should notice it and feel it, but not think about it. The goal is to try to be aware of the sensations your body is experiencing while you quiet the thinking part of the experience. Stay with this process for at least 10 minutes. If this feels excruciatingly long, do not be discouraged. Mindfulness is a skill that takes time to develop. Stick with it! Research shows that mindfulness meditation can actually change your brain. It seems that, with practice, meditation can activate the left side of the prefrontal cortex, the area associated with feelings of tranquility and joy (Goldin, Ramel, & Gross, 2009).

S.E.L.F. Care

Listen to those who tell you to take care of yourself. This cannot be emphasized enough. Things that seem way too obvious to be helpful can make the difference between a good and a bad day. Keep the acronym S.E.L.F. in mind to help you remember the important elements of self-care:

Sleep. Lack of sleep will make anxiety and depression worse. You might need to rearrange things or ask for help, but ensuring that you get a good night's sleep is essential to the management of distress. It goes without saying that the baby's sleep is intricately connected to your ability to get a good night's rest. Studies have shown that when infant sleep is problematic, sleep intervention strategies can benefit both baby and mother (Hiscock & Wake, 2001).

Exercise. Moving your body, even when you don't feel like it, can make a significant difference in the way you feel. Exercise can help diffuse the adrenaline produced by anxiety, ease muscle tension, and promote better sleep. It also enhances well-being by releasing endorphins, the chemicals in the brain associated with feeling good. Even though it is not easy to do when you are overwhelmed and overloaded, small steps can make a difference. A little bit of exercise is better than none. Exercise has been shown to improve levels of depression during the postpartum period (Armstrong &

Edwards, 2003), as well as to combat anxiety in general (DeMoor, Beem, Stubbe, Boomsma, & DeGeus, 2006). Therefore, it makes sense that exercise would also be beneficial in the management of scary thoughts. At a minimum, it will provide another source of distraction; at a maximum, it will stimulate endorphins that counteract the distress you are experiencing.

Laugh. It sounds like such a cliché that it seems it couldn't make a real difference. But it can. It feels good to laugh. Laughter exercises the abdominal muscles and lungs. During a hearty belly laugh, the heart rate increases quickly. This was demonstrated by Dr. William Fry, a pioneer in the research of laughter, who observed that after 1 minute of hearty laughter, his heart rate was equal to the rate he achieved after 10 minutes on a rowing machine (Fry, 1992). Several studies have demonstrated laughter's significant physiological impact on the body's immune system. Laughter has been shown to lower levels of adrenaline and cortisol—hormones that are released in times of stress—and to raise levels of endorphins (Berk et al., 1989). If you find that laughter is difficult for you, try a "half-smile," curving the corners of your mouth upward. Your facial expressions are hard-wired to your brain, so turning the corners of your mouth upward sends signals to the brain to feel good (Linehan, 1993).

Food. Modifying your diet can help reduce anxiety:

- Eating frequent small meals can help stabilize blood sugar. Swings in blood sugar can cause symptoms that mimic anxiety, such as light-headedness.
- Drink lots of water. It has been shown that dehydration can affect your mood (Hall-Flavin, 2009).
- Eating complex carbohydrates (whole grains) can increase serotonin, which is associated with feelings of calmness.
- Restrict simple carbohydrates (sugar).
- Increase your intake of fruit, vegetables, and fish. Decrease consumption of processed foods and high-fat dairy, which have been linked to higher levels of depression and anxiety (Jacka et al., 2010).
- Avoid alcohol.
- Avoid caffeine. Caffeine can exacerbate anxiety and interfere with sleep.

Journaling

Another self-help strategy that has proven to be useful is writing things down or journaling. Journaling can be an effective tool for self-examination and expression. However, a couple words of caution regarding the journaling experience are necessary. Some women report resistance to the notion of putting anything negative down in writing. Putting scary thoughts into words seems to give them more life for some women, thereby reinforcing them. Random venting can feel pointless and daunting. Other women become anxious at the thought of writing down scary thoughts because they are concerned that someone may find it, their child may read it years from now, or it may in some other way incriminate them.

If a woman is resistant due to these concerns, but the idea of writing appeals to her, Karen will ask her to buy a separate notebook for this purpose and bring it in with her to sessions. In this way, they can review the entries together, providing structure and purpose. It is up to the client whether she wants to rip out the pages and leave them with Karen or tear them up as a ritualistic gesture to free her from what she has written. Some women state that writing down their thoughts helps purge their scary thoughts, particularly when they bring them into a therapy session for validation and guidance. Whatever the process entails, the act of writing is encouraged only if it feels like a positive self-help intervention.

Self-Help Materials

The term *bibliotherapy* means to help through the use of books, but this term also extends to the use of other written materials, computer or Internet programs, and audio- or video-taped materials for addressing specific problems (Marrs, 1995). For our purposes, we will use the term *self-help materials* to incorporate all of these treatment options.

One major advantage of self-help materials is that you can read or view the information at your own pace and convenience. Postpartum women face many logistical challenges that can interfere with making and keeping appointments for professional intervention. You are already attending so many other appointments, such as your follow-up visits with your obstetrician and pediatrician. If you are home full-time with your child while your partner is at work, then you might have to think about child care arrangements while you are off at a doctor's appointment. If you have gone back to work, then you might need to juggle appointments with the demands of your job, the hours of your day care, and other obligations that you must meet during your off-work hours. Even if you are able to carve out some time to meet with a healthcare professional about your scary thoughts, you might simply be too tired or overwhelmed to attend when it is time to get in the car. You might decide that self-help materials and resources are a better option for you for these reasons.

Self-help materials are often simple and cost effective. In contrast, professional intervention often requires some investment of financial resources and time. Those who have insurance that covers mental health services may need to find a provider in their network and pay a copay for services at each visit. Some mental health providers do not accept insurance and require payment of their full fee for each visit. Those who do not have health insurance or whose health insurance does not cover mental health services often can find low-cost alternatives in the community (e.g., sliding-scale services at a training clinic or at a social services agency), but it may take time to research and locate these options.

Although this may be discouraging, keep in mind that sometimes the expense of intervention is far less of a consideration than long-term suffering. In this way, the cost of not seeking help when it is needed can be significantly greater. Even though you typically take care of everyone else before taking steps to care for yourself, the value of making your needs a priority at this critical time should not be undermined by cost or stigma. As you decide whether you would benefit from professional or nonprofessional intervention, we encourage you to explore the strategies in this chapter to determine what level of support is best for you.

The potential disadvantages to using self-help materials should be noted. First, the fact that a woman can access these materials at her leisure can be as much of a curse as it is a blessing. To be effective, they often require consistent attention and practice, which is challenging for a sleep-deprived mother whose baby's needs seem never ending. For a new mother who lacks energy and focus and the ability to sustain attention, reading might be the last thing she wants to add to her plate.

Another shortcoming is that these materials have rarely been evaluated in the research literature (Rosen, 1987), which means that there is little scientific evidence that, as a "treatment package," they successfully reduce scary thoughts and emotional distress above and beyond the passage of time. However, research on the effectiveness of the use of self-help resources for anxiety disorders suggests that, in general, they are more effective than not trying anything at all (Hirai & Clum, 2006; Newman, Erickson, Przeworski, & Dzus, 2003).

A good strategy for making self-help materials work for you is to set aside time to read or view them regularly and actively. These materials often suggest various exercises, and it is important to test them out on several occasions and evaluate their effectiveness before dismissing them. Self-help materials work for some people but not for others. Try some of the suggestions to see if something helps you feel better.

Support Groups

Support groups for women with postpartum anxiety or depression are useful in reducing the debilitating isolation of suffering alone. It can be enormously comforting to find others sharing common anxieties who can relate to the concerns you are having. Support groups help by normalizing and validating the experience each participant is having. An effective support group can help eliminate some of the myths surrounding scary thoughts by sharing personal experiences along with any relevant psychoeducational information. We include support groups in this section because they are often led by peers; however, some support groups are facilitated by mental health professionals. These are described in the next chapter.

The mechanisms that drive the success of many support groups are supportive listening, problem clarification, and problem-solving techniques (Milgrom, Negri, Gemmill, McNeil, & Martin, 2005). When these dynamics emerge within the framework of a group process, women report that they feel validated and deeply understood. Due to the overwhelming stigma and women's reticence toward reaching out to professionals, some women tell us they are most comfortable in support groups. Being surrounded by others who experience similar symptoms of anxiety can make scary thoughts feel less threatening.

However, the opposite can also be true: Some women find the group environment more threatening than an individual setting. Women who are more introverted by nature may feel uncomfortable expressing themselves in groups. Other women might mistakenly compare themselves to women in the group who seem to be doing a better job than they are at pretending that everything is fine, thereby "looking" better or healthier. This causes them to misconstrue that no other woman could possibly be experiencing the same awful thoughts that they are having In fact, some women have told us that they have left support groups feeling worse than they did before they went.

Some women may misinterpret what others are saying or have difficulty tolerating the anxiety of others while they are feeling so fragile. This is a fundamental hazard of unstructured groups and the reason why postpartum support groups that provide a structured format with predetermined topics of discussion are more successful. By focusing the groups in this way, women who are symptomatic can gain support and guidance with less risk of exposing themselves to increased anxiety.

If you are wondering whether a support group would be helpful to you, consider the following:

- The greater your level of distress and level of impairment are, the greater is the likelihood that professional intervention is needed.
- Your personal style and preferences will influence your comfort level in a group setting.

Still, remember not to place too much emphasis on any resistance you might have because your emotions are high right now, and you may need to push through some of your hesitation in order to benefit from the support of others.

The rewards derived from a support group are largely based on the nature of the supportive interactions. In particular, feeling understood and less isolated provides a great sense of control and empowerment, which leads to more effective ways of coping (Helgeson & Gottlieb, 2000). In fact, one study showed that the beneficial outcome and general satisfaction among members of support groups were equivalent to those of professionally provided, more expensive interventions (Pistrang, Barker, & Humphreys, 2008).

Online Support

The Internet has long held the promise of widespread access to abundant support outlets. Indeed, online support communities, where women experience virtual connections with others who share similar experiences, have rapidly become a rising form of social networking. These avenues of support include blogs, chat rooms, informational Web sites, interactive discussion forums or message boards, and newsgroups. New technology is increasing the popularity of social communication tools, such as Facebook, MySpace, Twitter, and LinkedIn, with more emerging all the time.

Online support communities can be invaluable, and the best advice is to start with paths that have been well traveled, such as Postpartum Progress (www.postpartumprogress.com), Postpartum Support International (postpartum.net), and The Postpartum Stress Center (postpartumstress. com). These are respected sites for postpartum women seeking online support and will also link directly to additional highly regarded resources.

One of the strengths of online support is the anonymity of the participant, which has been associated with greater disclosure of emotion (Miller, 2006). Research on the effects of online support is sparse; to our knowledge, nothing in the literature specifically addresses the efficacy of online support with regard to postpartum distress and scary thoughts. It is worth noting, however, that there is a great deal of descriptive and anecdotal affirmation of the popularity of online or virtual support communities. We frequently hear women report that their experience with online communities has been their greatest source of ongoing and unconditional support.

One additional cautionary note is that in the absence of such trustworthy sources, random searching and unmoderated peer-to-peer support can sometimes lead to misinformed voices or inaccurate information. As we might expect, misinformation regarding the presence and meaning of scary thoughts whirls through cyberspace. If a person is not careful, anxiety can erupt wildly at the very sight of one mistaken comment or erroneous bit of information. In the worst-case scenario, exposure to false information or fear-provoking exaggerations can cause women to recoil further into dangerous levels of retreat. It is recommended that postpartum women stay close to the postpartum sites mentioned earlier, which are careful to present the supportive and accurate information postpartum women are seeking.

Omega-3 Fatty Acids

In our culture's quest for health and happiness, a subject of recent attention has been the depletion of essential fatty acids, such as eicosapentaenoic (EPA) and docosahexaenoic (DHA) acids, from Western diets (Maes, Christophe, Delanghe, et al., 1999). These acids are referred to as essential because they cannot be synthesized by the human body and must be obtained from dietary sources. Some rich sources are fish, such as tuna, salmon, herring, and sardines, and certain plants, such as flaxseed, canola oil, and walnuts. Studies show that low levels of omega-3 fatty acids in the diet are associated with low levels of serotonin, which is linked with anxiety and depression (Freeman et al., 2008).

Although it should be acknowledged that omega-3 fatty acids have yet to be tested in the specific treatment of scary thoughts, experts now recommend the use of fish oil supplements as a safe treatment option for depression during both pregnancy and the postpartum period. Fish oil supplements seem to be well tolerated, with little or no adverse effects reported. A dosage of 1 or 2 grams daily has been shown to augment treatment with antidepressants (Nemets, Stahl, & Belmaker, 2002; Peet, Murphy, Shay, & Horrobin, 1998). Remember always to check with your physician for dosing instructions.

Light Therapy

Most often associated with the treatment of seasonal affective disorder, bright-light therapy, or exposure to artificial light, is another intervention that may be preferred by women who are interested in nonprofessional interventions. Studies have shown that the rate of production of serotonin (associated with mood) by the brain is directly related to the duration of bright sunlight and increases rapidly with increased exposure to light (Lambert, Reid, Kaye, Jennings, & Esler, 2002). The investment is small, typically around $200 for a portable light box that can be used in the comfort of the home.

In a small study of pregnant women with major depression, bright-light therapy produced antidepressant effects (Oren et al., 2002). Full-spectrum light boxes have also proven to be beneficial with postpartum depression (Corral, Kuan, & Kostaras, 2000). Though research is needed with regard to scary thoughts, experts agree that this is a favorable option for pregnant and postpartum women in distress because it is easily accessible, extremely well tolerated, and safe while breastfeeding. Light therapy involves a low-risk effort that enables you to carve out time in your morning to sit and take care of yourself. You can use the light box while you are at your computer or having a cup of coffee reading the morning paper. In this way, you will be augmenting your serotonin and finding precious time to relax at the same time.

UNDERSTANDING THE LARGER CONTEXT

Bear in mind that almost everything is exaggerated during the postpartum period: the environment, the body, relationships, social influences, sounds, smells. The entire milieu is intensely impacted, and each and every sensitive response is maximized. Most attempts to exert control over unruly and unfamiliar territory are met with opposition or disappointment. Understanding the sensitive nature of this tender time is an essential element of early acceptance. How does one accept something that feels so bad? Three suggestions follow.

Identify the Emotions

Scary thoughts make people extremely anxious. Although this may seem to be an obvious understatement, it is nonetheless important to reemphasize. The distress that accompanies scary thoughts serves as a reminder that these thoughts are inconsistent with the sufferer's sense of self and therefore do not signal a greater danger. This is not to say that the distress is unremarkable or is unresponsive to treatment. Quite the contrary, distress linked to scary thoughts can be debilitating and can range from avoidant behaviors all the way to the sense that one is losing one's mind. Identifying this emotional state as commonplace in such circumstances is important. Fear of the distress itself is a slippery slope because it can rapidly lead to more and more feelings of uncontrollable distress.

Acknowledge the Current State

There is power in acknowledging one's powerlessness. Great resiliency can be achieved when one is able to surrender to some extent and let go of secondary panic. It is natural to react with alarm when thoughts and feelings are scary and unsettling, but it is well established that when one fears the fear, distress escalates. In such situations, straightforward affirmations reflecting the current state can be helpful:

- I am having scary thoughts. I might not understand why this is happening, but I know it is common and it happens to many mothers.

- My scary thoughts are not me. They are either a symptom of OCD or PPD, or they are just a function of my anxiety right now. They will not always be here.
- I don't like the way it feels, but I am doing what I need to do to feel better.
- I understand that my anxiety is a natural part of becoming a mother, and even though it makes me feel terrible at times, I can endure it because I know I will not always feel this way.

Acceptance

Asking an exhausted, overwhelmed mother to work toward accepting the presence of a negative emotional experience can feel like an imposing task. But consider the words of psychoanalyst Carl Jung (1932): "We cannot change anything unless we accept it. Condemnation does not liberate, it oppresses" (Chang, 2006, p. 24). As the concept of mindfulness teaches us, acceptance does not mean liking the scary thoughts. Rather, it means believing, at least for the time being, that they exist, and understanding that they may be there whether one likes it or not.

The reason why acceptance is such an important step is that it sets in motion the appropriate responses, such as letting go, which are less likely to cause rebounding scary thoughts. The inability to accept what is happening will lead to misguided efforts to control what cannot be controlled. Without a doubt, all of the barriers discussed in Chapter 5, as well as countless additional irrational distortions, are blocks to acceptance. Accepting anxiety and scary thoughts is not easy. It takes more effort for some than for others. But it will, indeed, reduce scary thoughts and lessen distress over them, so it's a challenge worth taking.

How can we simplify this task? You need to acknowledge that this is happening. Remember that no harm will come as a result of these scary thoughts. Understand that they will pass whether you are in a situation that requires treatment or not. Observe as your anxiety goes up and down. Rate your feelings of distress between 0 and 10 (with 10 being the highest level). Be aware that a 6 on the distress scale may not feel as good as a 0, but it's substantially better than the way a 9 feels!

Learn to breathe while you try to move from a 6 down to a 5. Understand that during this fragile time, the distress will continue to fluctuate. When it goes up again, recognize that this is how anxiety manifests, and see if you can bring it down just a notch. The mistake women often make is that they want it gone completely. They want feelings of distress to go from an 8 to a 0. Remember that anxiety occurs on a continuum—it's not black and white, anxious or not anxious. It goes up and it comes down. Then it goes up again. Accept that this is happening. If you pay attention to the rise and fall, you can make incremental changes that lessen the distress.

The Six Points is a tool that was developed to help manage symptoms of anxiety (Zane, 1984, p. 242). We find these simple directives to be a compelling reminder to women who are constantly plagued by distress. Copy these points down and keep them with you. The more you practice them when you anticipate anxiety or feel anxious, the more you will see how they work to ease your discomfort:

THE SIX POINTS

1. Expect, allow, and accept that fear will arise.
2. When fear comes, stop, wait, and let it be.
3. Focus on and do manageable things in the present.
4. Label your level of fear from 0 to 10. Watch it go up and down.
5. Function with fear. Appreciate your achievements.
6. Expect, allow, and accept fear reappearing.

Letting Go and Letting In

Michel de Montaigne (n.d.), a sixteenth-century French writer, said, "Nothing fixes a thing so intensely in the memory as the wish to forget it." Here, again, we see the paradox that is so ever present in any discussion of negative thoughts. Our very desire to make them go away often makes them feel more potent. It is an unkind twist to an instinctively protective mechanism.

How do you let go? This is a concept that attracts a great deal of attention in pop psychology circles: letting go of your past, letting go of grudges, letting go of clutter, letting go of your emancipating children, letting go of a lost love. The list is endless. The concept of letting go generally refers to the combination of two things: (a) accepting the presence of some current (perhaps painful) state, and (b) forgiving or embracing your accountability and vulnerability within that state.

Think of it like this: Something is happening that causes stress (e.g., children leaving for college). In response to this event, there is something or nothing that you can do. If something should or could be done to relieve that stress, action needs to take place, (i.e., taking an evening class or reconnecting with friends). However, if action would not be helpful, then you need to learn to adapt to this new state of being (i.e., empty nest). This process of learning to let go needs to take place when no direct action is necessary, but relief from emotional distress is sought. Sometimes doing nothing is the hardest thing of all to do.

Ironically, the concept of doing nothing or taking no action with regard to emotional adjustment is one that requires much work. It necessitates a desire to transcend the mired state of current discomfort and let go in order to move forward. Spiritual teacher and author Eckhard Tolle (1999) uses a simple metaphor that helps elucidate this complicated process in responding to a question that he is frequently asked:

> How do we drop negativity? By dropping it. How do you drop a piece of hot coal you are holding in your hand? How do you drop some heavy and useless baggage that you are carrying? By recognizing that you don't want to suffer or carry the burden anymore and then letting go of it. (Tolle, 1999, p. 79)

This is an example of how simple something so complicated can be. Karen finds the use of this image most helpful when used in conjunction with a sound bite and gesture. Vocalizing the words *hot coal*, coinciding with a hand motion from a closed fist to an open one, can signal the brain that it should "let go." Believe it or not, our brains learn to respond appropriately when we train them in this way. Imagine the hot coal burning the palm of your hand. Think of the pain that a scary thought can carry with it. Look at your hand, and feel the burn of that thought, and drop it. Next time the scary thought pops into your head, say, "hot coal," pop open your hand, and let go.

This concept of letting go has a related component that might feel equally difficult at first: letting in. In this context, *letting in* refers to a duality of trust—trusting yourself and the capacity of others to help you, while *not* trusting your impulse to deal with this on your own. Secrets have huge power, especially those that relate to taboo subjects. As we've seen, feelings of embarrassment and fear of disapproval can contribute to upholding the secret of scary thoughts. Postpartum women who are struggling with scary thoughts need to believe in the strength that comes from connection and open themselves to the solace that can come from trusting others to help. Reaching out at a time when all feels lost can be the single most beneficial step you can take.

High levels of distress and the accompanying scary thoughts can ambush even the most well prepared postpartum woman. One thing that we know for sure is that anxiety feels worse when you believe you are powerless. In this chapter, we explored ways for you to recalibrate some of your automatic response patterns and apply self-help strategies so that you can begin to break free from the grip of your scary thoughts. In the next chapter, you will learn concrete tools that have been proven to make a significant difference in decreasing anxiety associated with scary thoughts by directly targeting the thoughts themselves.

Take-Home Point for Mothers. The self-help strategies and nonprofessional interventions discussed here are not just things you can do to start to feel better. They are tried and true interventions that have been proven to make a significant difference in the course of anxiety and depressive symptoms and can help reduce the impact of the scary thoughts you are having. They will be useful whether you apply them on their own or in conjunction with professional support. If you're not sure whether the best option for you is using self-help, trying nonprofessional options, or seeking professional help, we encourage you to weigh the following factors:

- The degree to which your scary thoughts cause life interference and emotional distress
- The degree to which your symptoms might interfere with benefiting from self-help strategies (e.g., lack of concentration)
- Logistics (e.g., availability of child care, health insurance, time to research mental health clinicians)
- The degree to which any of these treatments have been helpful for you in the past

If your symptoms cause significant life interference and distress, and you find little or no benefit from self-help or nonprofessional interventions, then a professional treatment approach might be a better choice for you.

Clinician Note. Encouraging a postpartum woman to engage in self-help strategies will augment her feelings of control during this unpredictable time, as well as provide relief from some of her distress. Helping her to discover ways she can feel good again, even for short moments in time, will enable her to reclaim her self-esteem and offer the sweet taste of hopefulness.

8

Can You Really Change
How You Think?

We've seen that you can use a number of strategies to begin to ease the distress associated with your scary thoughts. As in the previous chapter, this chapter contains self-help strategies that have the potential to assist you in managing scary thoughts on your own. All of the techniques described in this chapter fall in the category of *cognitive* self-help strategies: These strategies target thinking, reasoning, and remembering.

Scary thoughts are cognitive in nature in that they involve verbal thoughts, visual images, and/or intrusive memories. It makes sense, then, that cognitive self-help strategies would be useful in reducing the frequency, intensity, and severity of scary thoughts. In this chapter, you will learn how to determine whether your scary thoughts are accurate and helpful or not. If you determine that they are not, you will discover how to modify them so that they are more balanced and evoke less distress. All of these cognitive strategies are often incorporated into cognitive behavioral therapy (CBT), which is described in Chapter 9. As a reminder, Chapter 11 provides space for you to make note of which strategies you have found most helpful and why.

WHY FOCUS ON THINKING?

Cognitive self-help strategies are based on the simple premise that the thoughts, images, beliefs, and other cognitions that people experience have a substantial effect on how they feel, which in turn can affect their behavior. Figure 8.1 summarizes this cognitive model. According to this model, when people experience certain *situations,* thoughts and images called *automatic thoughts* pop into their minds. The thoughts are described as automatic because they often come about so quickly that people are not fully aware that they have them. Nevertheless, automatic thoughts are often associated with distinct *emotions,* such as anxiety, sadness, or frustration. On the basis of these automatic thoughts and emotions, people choose a particular course of action or *behavior.* If their automatic thoughts are negatively biased, then it follows that they would experience negative emotions and that they might even choose a course of action that perpetuates these negative thoughts and emotions.

Consider two mothers of 6-week-old infants who find themselves in the same situation. Their babies are not getting enough milk from breastfeeding and therefore are not growing as much as is expected. Both women are faced with their physicians' recommendation of having to give up breast feeding and switch to bottle-feeding.

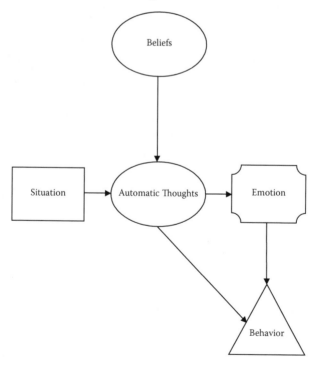

FIGURE 8.1
The cognitive model.

The first mother, Katherine, disliked breastfeeding from the beginning and experienced it as painful and uncomfortable. When she found herself in this situation, her first thoughts were, *Thank goodness. I'm grateful to have another feeding option that will work better for me and for the baby.* As a result, she experienced a sense of relief, and she immediately complied with her doctor's recommendation. Soon thereafter, her baby started growing rapidly because she was getting all the nutrition she needed; Katherine began to look forward to feeding the baby, rather than dreading it.

The second mother, Julie, had her heart set on breastfeeding well before the baby was born. All of her friends with children breastfed their babies, and she had thoroughly prepared for breastfeeding by taking classes, reading two books, and joining a lactation group. When her doctor recommended that she switch to bottle-feeding, her first thoughts were, *This is the worst possible scenario. Now my baby won't be healthy because he won't have the benefit of breast milk. And we won't have a strong bond. I've failed as a mother.* Not surprisingly, Julie experienced a great deal of sadness and despair. She was reluctant to give up breastfeeding, but was forced to do so as her baby continued to fall short of the growth progress her doctor thought essential. Soon thereafter, she avoided the phone calls and e-mail messages from other mothers in her lactation group.

There is an important message from these two contrasting examples: Two people can be faced with the same situation, but because they think about the situation in very different ways, they have very different emotional and behavioral reactions. In other words, it is not always a situation that causes a person to feel a certain way, but instead it is the manner in which the person perceives it or thinks about it. In many instances, people cannot fully change situations that life throws in their paths, but they *can* change how they think about them. This chapter will give you some ideas for ways to go about doing this.

Notice that one other construct in Figure 8.1 has not yet been discussed: *beliefs*. Beliefs are represented in an oval just like automatic thoughts because beliefs are another type of cognition. However, they are different from automatic thoughts because they are ideas to which people hold tightly regardless of the situation. Beliefs can be about oneself, about others, about the way the world works, or about the future. They are included in the cognitive model in Figure 8.1 because they often influence the types of automatic thoughts that arise in specific situations.

Katherine, for example, had a number of adaptive beliefs about herself and motherhood, such as: *Not everything will go perfectly, but I will be a good mother. It will all work out in the long run.* These beliefs are considered adaptive because they help her to adjust to the uncertainty of parenting a newborn and keep "bumps in the road" in perspective. When Katherine's doctor recommended that she discontinue breast feeding, she was understandably disappointed. She was better able to look on the positive side because she had not had a good experience with breast feeding.

In contrast, Julie operated under a different set of beliefs, and one of these beliefs was that *all good mothers breast feed.* This belief had the potential to be less adaptive than Katherine's beliefs because it set a high, rigid standard with the potential to be associated with great disappointment, guilt, and shame if it was not realized. Not surprisingly, when her doctor recommended that she discontinue breast feeding much earlier than she had expected, Julie experienced automatic thoughts in the form of excessive worry (*Now my baby won't be healthy because he won't have the benefit of breast milk*) and rumination (*I've failed as a mother*). This latter example demonstrates that all of the scary thoughts described in this book are examples of automatic thoughts. For the remainder of this chapter, the terms automatic thoughts and scary thoughts will be used interchangeably.

All of the cognitive strategies discussed here are applicable to automatic thoughts that arise in particular situations as well as tightly held beliefs. We recommend that you start with applying the strategies to automatic thoughts because they are more easily identified and modified. Over time, you should see a pattern to your automatic thoughts that will help you better understand your underlying beliefs. Modifying unwanted automatic thoughts will likely bring about reduction in your distress. However, the most lasting change will come from identifying and modifying any tightly held beliefs that give rise to upsetting automatic thoughts over and over again.

COGNITIVE SELF-HELP STRATEGIES

Identifying and Evaluating Scary Thoughts

The most basic way to modify scary thoughts is to learn how to identify and evaluate them. Then, after you examine them, you can determine whether or not they need to be altered so that they are more balanced. The word *balance* is important here; the goal of cognitive strategies is not simply thinking positively or thinking the opposite of the scary thought. In many cases, thinking positively or thinking the opposite can be just as unrealistic as the scary thought.

Instead, the goal is to take into consideration all the pieces of information, both good and bad, that pertain to the scary thought you are having and then construct a new statement that takes all of this information into account. Although some grains of the negative still might be in the new, more balanced thought, there should be enough non-negatives that the intensity of your distress will decrease to a reasonable level. This will help you to be more centered, take care of yourself, and choose reasonable courses of action to address whatever problems you are facing.

Step 1. Identify Scary Thoughts

When you notice a negative change in your mood (e.g., you feel more anxious or sad), try to identify the automatic thought that is associated with your emotion. Remember the cognitive model presented in Figure 8.1; emotional experiences stem, in large part, from the manner in which we perceive or think about situations in which people find themselves. So if you are experiencing a negative emotion, it is likely that it is tied to a negative automatic thought. The most central question to ask yourself is, *What thought was running through my mind in that situation?*

Because automatic thoughts, as their name states, are automatic, the task of answering this question is often easier said than done. When you first start this exercise, you might need to spend more time figuring out exactly what scary thought is causing you distress. Other questions that can help you target the specific scary thought are as follows:

- What do I believe was running through my mind in that situation?
- When I experienced similar situations in the past, what thoughts were running through my mind?
- Is it possible that I am focusing on a mental image or an intrusive memory, rather than a verbal thought?
- What does this situation really mean to me?

Even if you have to guess the content of your automatic thought on the basis of these questions, rather than pinpoint the precise thought, you will still gain valuable experience from this exercise because you will get practice in identifying the thoughts and this will be helpful in the long run.

To see how this works, go back to the case descriptions presented in Chapter 1. Each of the women described in that chapter experienced some sort of automatic thought that caused her distress.

- Amanda, the mother described on p. 9, who engaged in excessive worry, reported automatic thoughts such as: *It feels like I will never sleep through the night again* and *I'm imprisoned by my own life.*
- Lori, the mother described on p. 12, who engaged in rumination, reported automatic thoughts such as: *I'm such a loser* and *they will be better off without me.*
- Elizabeth, the mother described on p. 13, who reported obsessive thoughts, experienced many of her automatic thoughts in the form of images. Examples were mental pictures of her baby not breathing and of her older child falling over the edge of the wall of a parking garage.
- Angie, the mother described on p. 14, who had a traumatic childbirth, also experienced automatic thoughts as mental images. However, unlike Elizabeth, her mental images took the form of past memories, such as the doctor saying, "He's not breathing."
- Stephanie, the mother described on p. 16, experienced uncomfortable physical sensations and misinterpreted them as being catastrophes. (*Something is horribly wrong with my lungs; I'm going to die of lung cancer.*) These catastrophic misinterpretations can also be thought of as automatic thoughts and subjected to the analysis that is described in this section.

Table 8.1, the Scary Thought Log, provides a place to record your automatic thoughts and begin the process of evaluation. The first three columns correspond to the cognitive model, where you can note the situation, automatic thought, and emotion. For now, practice working with these three columns until you feel that you can identify the most central automatic thoughts that are causing distress.

We have three suggestions as you begin the process of identifying your automatic thoughts. First, it's okay if there is not necessarily an external situation that triggers an automatic thought. Many mothers indicate that

TABLE 8.1

Scary Thought Log

Situation	Thought	Emotion	Question the Thought	Balanced Response
• What triggered the scary thought?	• What thought(s) ran through your mind? • What do you guess was running through your mind? • What thoughts did you experience in similar situations in the past? • What did the situation mean to you?	• What feeling(s) did you experience?	• What evidence supports the scary thought? • What evidence against the scary thought? • What is the realistic likelihood that _____ will happen?	• After questioning the scary thought, what is the most balanced way of viewing this situation? • How can I account for all of the information that goes into the way I am looking at this situation?

their scary thoughts come out of the blue, such as when they are trying to fall asleep. If this is the case, write *Thought came out of the blue when I was* _____ in your Scary Thought Log. You might even find that an internal experience triggers a scary thought, such as another thought (e.g., wondering what it will be like when you start your baby at day care), an emotion (e.g., nervous), or a physical sensation (e.g., heart racing), rather than an external experience.

Second, it is likely that you will experience a number of scary thoughts and find it difficult to sort them out. You are encouraged to write down as many thoughts as you think are relevant. It is best, though, to record the thoughts that are most central to your emotional distress, which often can be identified when you ask yourself, *What does this situation mean to me?*

Third, it is most effective to complete the Scary Thought Log soon after you notice the automatic thought. The reason for this is so that you can capture the thoughts and emotions as accurately as possible before other things in life intervene and the situation resolves itself. However, if it's too much trouble to do this, given the demands of caring for a newborn, set aside time during the day when you can complete the Scary Thought Log all at once.

Step 2: Question the Scary Thoughts

The best way to get perspective on automatic thoughts is to ask yourself questions that lead to their critical evaluation and to do your best to answer those questions as thoroughly and thoughtfully as possible. The following are questions you might find helpful to ask yourself as you begin to get perspective on your scary thoughts (Beck, 1995; Wiegartz & Gyoerkoe, 2009):

- What evidence do I have that supports the scary thought? What evidence do I have that does not support the scary thought?
- Do I know for certain that_____ will happen?
- What is the realistic likelihood that _____ will happen?
- What is the most likely outcome?
- If something bad happens, how will I handle it? Have I been able to handle adversity in the past?
- How often have I been correct when I have predicted the worst-case scenario in the past?
- Does _____ have to lead to _____?

- Could there be any other reasons why _____ is happening? What are those reasons?
- How useful is it for me to be focusing on this scary thought right now?
- What negative consequences are there for focusing on this scary thought right now?
- What would I tell a friend if she were experiencing the same scary thought?

Although these are some of the most common questions we use in our clinical practices, you do not have to be limited to this list. In fact, the more personalized the questions are for your circumstances, the more compelling the questions will be to you, and the more you will be able to evaluate the automatic thought as realistically as possible.

Let's take a closer look at how this works with the examples presented previously. Notice that each of the mothers chose some of the standard questions listed here, as well as others that were modified to fit her particular circumstances:

- To evaluate the automatic thought it feels like I will never sleep through the night again, Amanda asked herself, What is the realistic likelihood that I will never sleep through the night again? Isn't it normal for mothers of newborns to feel sleep deprived? To evaluate the automatic thought I'm imprisoned in my own life, Amanda asked herself, Is it really useful to be thinking about my situation by using terms like "imprisoned"? Is this way of viewing my life just making it all the more unbearable?
- To evaluate the automatic thought I'm such a loser, Lori asked herself, What evidence supports the idea that I am a loser? What things in my life have I done that suggest the opposite, that I am not a loser? To evaluate the automatic thought they will be better off without me, Lori asked herself, What would be the realistic consequences of my leaving? How would my leaving hurt my family?
- To gain perspective on the obsessive images of death coming to her children, Elizabeth asked herself, What is the realistic likelihood that something this bad would happen? Aren't there signs I will notice in advance before these tragedies would occur?

- To gain perspective on the intrusive memories of the doctor saying that her baby wasn't breathing, Angie asked herself, Is there any truth to that statement now? Isn't my baby okay now?
- To evaluate her catastrophic misinterpretations of uncomfortable physical sensations, Stephanie asked herself, Could there be any other reasons that I am experiencing these sensations? How many times have I experienced these sensations in the past, only to find that nothing medically is wrong with me?

The fourth column in the Scary Thought Log is a place for you to record one or two questions that you think will be particularly helpful to gain perspective and balance regarding these thoughts. Each time you write down these questions, you increase the probability that they will come up just as automatically as the scary thoughts in the future. In fact, we anticipate that you will not have to record your scary thoughts on the log long term. As you become practiced in identifying and questioning your automatic thoughts, the process will come easily to you, and you will be able to apply these strategies as soon as you notice a scary thought.

Step 3: Construct a Balanced Response

Asking the questions described in the previous section is crucial for the final step in the process: constructing a more accurate response to the automatic thought that reflects balance, perspective, and insight. You will take this step if, after critically evaluating your scary thought, you determine that it is inaccurate or exaggerated. At times, you might conclude that a scary thought is indeed realistic. However, it will still be in your best interest to construct a balanced response because focusing on the thought is unhelpful and only causes more distress.

A balanced response incorporates the answers to the questions that you pose to yourself. It is often a bit lengthier than the automatic thought so that it reflects the positives, negative, and neutral aspects of the situation. The trick is to compose a balanced response that is as compelling as possible so that you ultimately put more stock in it than in the scary thought. The following are examples of the balanced responses constructed by the mothers we have been considering throughout this section:

- Amanda's balanced responses: (a) It is true that sleep deprivation does not feel good. But most mothers go through this, and they somehow survive it. I am fortunate that I am still on maternity leave and do not need to be in tip-top shape to function at work. (b) Viewing myself as being imprisoned only makes things worse. Although I am the primary caretaker of the baby, I am going to be mindful of the relief that I get from my husband and mother.
- Lori's balanced responses: (a) Most mothers of newborns have trouble adjusting to parenthood; there isn't any reason why that makes me more of a loser than any of those other mothers. And, I have done plenty of things in my life to be proud of, like getting a graduate degree and having a good career. (b) Realistically, leaving would hurt the family much more than would staying. My husband would think I don't care about him; he would have to take care of our baby all on his own, and our baby would grow up without a mother.
- Elizabeth's balanced response: The likelihood of horrible tragedies happening to my kids is extremely low. There almost certainly will be signs in advance that I will see and can do something about. I have to remember that there is a lot of uncertainty associated with raising children and that I can't control everything.
- Angie's balanced response: It is okay to acknowledge that the baby's delivery was traumatic for me. But my baby IS breathing now, and he is healthy and happy. There's nothing about the delivery that can affect the baby now.
- Stephanie's balanced response: There are plenty of reasonable explanations for my difficulty breathing, especially the fact that I am out of shape. I have called the doctor when I have gotten scared about my physical symptoms five times now, and, in each instance, there was nothing medically wrong with me. The most likely reality is that nothing is wrong with me now.

See if you can now record the balanced responses to your own scary thoughts in the fifth column of the Scary Thought Log. Pay attention to the outcome of constructing the balanced response. Has the negative emotion that you recorded in the third column of the log decreased? Are you experiencing any new emotions, such as relief or hopefulness? Or, might you be prepared to do something differently, like letting others look after the baby while you take a much needed break? Noticing a positive or adaptive outcome from completing this exercise should reassure you that the exercise is effective.

Don't be discouraged if you do not discern a positive or adaptive outcome right away. This process takes practice, and it is unrealistic to think that the use of the Scary Thought Log once or twice will eliminate the automatic thoughts and the distress that they cause. If, even after you practice, this process doesn't seem effective for you, we have a few suggestions. First, you might take a close look at the automatic thoughts that you list in the second column of the log. Are they really the most central scary thoughts that are causing you distress? Try to challenge yourself to identify the fundamental meaning associated with the scary thoughts.

Second, you might also take a close look at the balanced responses you have constructed. Are they really compelling? Do they address all of the issues associated with your scary thoughts, or do they leave some issues unanswered? Would there be a question that would be a better match as you gain perspective on the scary thought?

Third, although some women are very much attracted to the logical, step-by-step analysis that the Scary Thought Log allows, other women find it artificial and removed from real life. In these cases, different approaches to modifying unhelpful automatic thoughts are indicated, as described in the following sections.

Experiments

Sometimes the most powerful information that can change a viewpoint comes from firsthand experience. It is one thing to evaluate the accuracy and helpfulness of automatic thoughts on paper using a thought log; it is another thing to test the accuracy and helpfulness of automatic thoughts in our own environments and observe the degree to which they are valid. Results from these real-life "experiments" often provide the most convincing evidence that can, in turn, make up a balanced response.

Consider Elizabeth's obsessive thoughts about her newborn stopping breathing. In addition to upsetting images of this occurring, Elizabeth also held the belief that if she did not check on her baby every 15 minutes, she would miss any signs of danger and her baby would die. As a result, she slept only in fits and starts and was chronically sleep deprived. Through the use of the Scary Thought Log she realized that it was unrealistic to think that checking on her baby that frequently would prevent a tragedy, but she could not bring herself to fully believe and act on that balanced response.

To examine this scary thought further, Elizabeth constructed an experiment in which she allowed herself to check on her baby on her own accord on only one occasion—halfway through the night; she could only check on her baby on other occasions if she heard the baby crying on the baby monitor. She recorded the number of times she checked on her baby and how she felt in the morning, and she compared these values to similar data she collected when she was using her old strategy of checking on her baby every 15 minutes.

Elizabeth learned that she checked on her baby four times throughout the night, using the new strategy, and over 20 times during the night using her old strategy. She also learned that she felt much more rested and energized when she used the new strategy. Most importantly, she learned that checking on the baby every 15 minutes was unnecessary and, in fact, was probably detrimental to her own well-being because she was so sleep deprived that it was difficult for her to stay calm and centered during the day when she was alone with her children. Thus, after conducting the experiment, Elizabeth now fully believed the balanced response that there was little, if any, likelihood that something would happen to her baby if she did not check on her every 15 minutes.

Not all of the scary thoughts that you experience will be amenable to testing through experiments. Another one of Elizabeth's intrusive visual images occurred when her son ran toward the wall of a parking garage. Clearly, she would err on the side of caution and would not experiment with letting him run to the edge without close supervision. However, if you have the sense that your scary thoughts are exaggerated and it would be safe to conduct an experiment, we would encourage you to do so and then use the information you gather in refining your balanced response.

Coping Cards

We recognize that the demands of parenting a newborn are great and that on many days you do not have time to grab a shower or have a healthy meal, let alone complete a full entry on the Scary Thought Log. Coping cards are a quick and easy way to reap some of the same benefits of the thought log exercise. You can record helpful information to put scary thoughts in perspective on an index card, business card, or even a piece of paper and have it readily available to consult in times of acute distress. The more you read your coping card when you experience a scary thought, the more you will be reminded of a more balanced approach to viewing your situation.

Coping cards can take many forms. Some women experience one primary scary thought that runs over and over in their mind. In these cases, they could construct a coping card in which they write the scary thought on one side and the balanced response on the other side. Angie took this approach; on one side of her coping card, she wrote, *memory of the doctor saying that the baby wasn't breathing.* On the other side, she wrote, *it is okay to acknowledge that the baby's delivery was traumatic for me. But the baby IS breathing now, and he is healthy and happy. There's nothing about the delivery that can affect the baby now.*

Other women find it helpful to generate a list of evidence that refutes their scary thoughts. For example, Lori found that the balanced response to her automatic thought, *I'm such a loser,* reduced her distress in some but not all instances. To bring a greater degree of perspective to this automatic thought, on her coping card she listed 10 reasons that did not support the idea that she is a loser. This strategy ensured that she did not forget any of the evidence that was contrary to her automatic thought.

Coping cards are useful in reducing the intensity of negative emotions and can be used to prompt some of the strategies described in the previous chapter. Because Amanda worried about so many things, she found it difficult to construct a coping card that captured all of the thoughts that ran through her mind. She elected to construct a coping card that contained two encouraging self-statements. On one side, she wrote, *just breathe. This moment will pass.* On the other side, she recorded an inspirational quotation from her favorite poet. Although these statements might not have helped her to modify any one scary thought, they helped her to gain perspective on the distress she was having in the moment and the larger difficulty she was having as she adjusted to motherhood.

Coping cards can also be used to summarize the self-help strategies that are most helpful and commonly used in one place, so that they are easily accessible in times of distress. Stephanie made a coping card that listed a combination of the strategies from this and the previous chapter that she found most helpful, including two ways to distract herself, a reminder to use controlled breathing, and two of the questions that could help her gain perspective on her scary thoughts.

Discussion With a "Coach"

Some women find that writing about a scary thought is too abstract and that it is more useful to apply the strategies described in this chapter in a verbal format. Identifying and evaluating scary thoughts with another person can be helpful in that this individual can work beside you to determine the most important scary thoughts to evaluate, the best questions to ask to gain perspective, and the most compelling balanced responses. In essence, this person can serve as a "coach" to encourage and help you when you need support. In addition, going through this process out loud can be an effective tool for ensuring that these strategies sink in and can be recalled on a later occasion.

You might have mixed feelings about adopting certain people as your coach. It will not be helpful to you if the person you hope will coach you merely tells you to "get over it" or gives you a balanced response without allowing you to grapple with the process. The key is for the two of you to read the strategies described in this chapter together and to work collaboratively to implement them in a step-by-step manner.

If this is a person whom you are around a great deal, then he or she can prompt you to apply the strategies in instances in which you experience a scary thought. If this is a person whom you don't see very often, then perhaps you can arrange to talk to him or her from time to time via telephone. Having a regular "check-in" will hold you accountable, reinforce the use of these strategies, and allow an opportunity to obtain care and support from a trusted individual. Not only will this achieve the aim of acquiring the cognitive strategies described in this chapter, but it also will allow you to make good use of a social support.

PUTTING IT ALL TOGETHER

The strategies described in this chapter directly target the identification, evaluation, and modification of scary thoughts. They are based on the cognitive behavioral approach to treatment that has been shown to be effective countless times in the research literature on anxiety disorders and depression. Although they might seem difficult or artificial at first, we are hopeful that, with some creativity and perseverance, you will be able to find the best combination to help you to achieve a balanced response to your scary thoughts. Remember that the strategies might seem awkward at first and you will need to spend time simply identifying scary thoughts when they arise. Then, work on questioning them and then on constructing balanced responses.

These strategies are meant to be used in conjunction with those described in the previous chapter. For example, some women find that it is easiest to focus on the Scary Thought Log only after they engage in a breathing or relaxation exercise. Other women find that these cognitive strategies reduce their emotional distress enough to engage in distraction or journaling. The important point is that you try the strategies described in the book and then determine what works best for you. Chapter 11 will help you to develop your personalized treatment plan on the basis of your practice with these techniques.

Take-Home Point for Mothers. Cognitive strategies help you to take a step back from your scary thoughts, evaluate whether they are helpful and accurate, and achieve balance and perspective. With practice, when you apply these strategies you may find that they can change your thinking.

Clinician Note. The strategies described in this chapter are standard techniques used by cognitive behavioral therapists who treat clients with anxiety and depression. Although these strategies have been shown to reduce emotional distress, we caution you against suggesting or applying them without thought given to the larger postpartum context in which the woman currently finds herself. These strategies are most effective when coupled with validation, compassion, and support from close others in their lives and healthcare professionals.

9

Professional Treatment Options

As mentioned in Chapter 4, the last thing you want to think about is making a decision about what to do to feel better. Everything is harder during this time. Trying to determine what course of action to take, when you are feeling unhinged by too many options already, can feel impossible. In Chapter 4, we outlined the criteria associated with various psychiatric disorders that can underlie scary thoughts to provide a context for the symptoms that you are experiencing. We also indicated that two main factors contribute to whether or not you are experiencing a psychiatric disorder and whether or not you decide to seek professional help: (a) the degree to which scary thoughts interfere with your life, and (b) the degree to which scary thoughts are distressing for you. Now that you have a sense of the degree to which your scary thoughts are associated with life interference and distress, we can weigh the advantages and disadvantages of various treatment options.

In Chapter 7, we discussed a variety of self-help strategies and nonprofessional interventions. In the following sections, we describe the professional treatment options (i.e., psychotherapy, medications). Professional options may be indicated if self-help strategies and/or nonprofessional interventions do not provide adequate relief. However, keep in mind that you do not have to choose one or the other. You can pursue a combination of the options described in Chapters 7 and 8 and those in this chapter if they feel right to you. If you find you are hesitant to consider professional treatment options, it may be helpful to find a dependable and knowledgeable support person with whom you can discuss these options.

PSYCHOTHERAPY

Often, going to therapy is not at the top of the list of things a postpartum woman wants to do. Karen noted in *Therapy and the Postpartum Woman:*

> While we underscore the notion that a postpartum woman may not be interested in therapy, we shift our focus to what she *does* want. Symptom relief. Pure and simple. That's it. She does not want to talk about how feelings of abandonment might be contributing to her sense of inadequacy. Nor does she want to explore how her impaired relationship with her mother might have impacted her self-esteem. She wants to sleep, to think clearly, to feel less anxious, and to stop crying all day. She wants to return to her previous level of functioning so she can get on with the business in her life. (Kleiman, 2008, p. 21)

Psychotherapy is an intervention that consists of the interaction between a mental health professional and a client who seeks help for emotional distress and/or current life difficulties. The objective of therapy is to improve her sense of well-being by providing support, developing a therapeutic relationship, and helping her acquire coping strategies. Not surprisingly, studies show that postpartum women tend to prefer psychotherapy over medication, especially if they are breastfeeding (Pearlstein et al., 2006). It's important to note here that there is reasonable evidence to support the use of psychotherapy as a stand-alone, first-line intervention for the treatment of various degrees of postpartum distress, even for severe depression (Stuart, O'Hara, & Gorman, 2003). Thus, even if it's difficult to reconcile the need for therapy during a time when there is great pressure to feel tremendous joy about being a mother, sometimes it can be imperative.

As we've discussed, by and large, postpartum women are not always thrilled to enter into a therapeutic relationship at a time they are feeling hard pressed to find the hours or the energy to do even the most routine tasks. In addition to the logistical constraints, therapy can be perceived as an indulgence, an unnecessary obligation, or an expensive waste of time. But therapy works. It works in ways that reduce negative feelings and scary thoughts and that, ultimately, help women feel better. In this section, we discuss the most common and well-documented therapies for the treatment of postpartum anxiety and depression: (a) supportive, (b) cognitive behavioral, (c) interpersonal, and (d) group therapy.

Supportive Psychotherapy

Most of the research with pregnant and postpartum women focuses on the efficacy of cognitive behavioral therapy and interpersonal therapy (Pearlstein et al., 2006), both of which are described in the sections that follow. Supportive psychotherapy has received far less attention in the general literature, yet it is probably the therapy most often used by clinicians who practice in this field. One study found that supportive psychotherapy and pharmacotherapy (the use of medication as treatment) were equally effective and suggested that patients and therapists prefer supportive psychotherapy over pharmacotherapy with respect to the reduction of depressive symptoms (DeMaat et al., 2008). We describe supportive psychotherapy before other approaches to psychotherapy because many elements of supportive psychotherapy, such as empathy and a strong therapeutic relationship, are critical to the success of other types of psychotherapy.

Generally speaking, supportive psychotherapy is characterized by reflective listening and the expression and tolerance of affect, with an overall goal of improving the quality of one's life (Markowitz, Manber, & Rosen, 2008). Supportive psychotherapy can escort a postpartum woman toward better functioning by providing encouragement and guidance for her to bolster her adaptive skills. As many readers know from experience, it is a conversation-based therapy that uses direct approaches, such as praise, advice, clarification, confrontation, and interpretation (Rosenthal, Muran, Pinsker, Hellerstein, & Winston, 1999). Specifically, the therapist might summarize or paraphrase what is being said to let the woman know she is being heard and understood, or the therapist might bring attention to an issue that the woman might be avoiding. These techniques are especially comforting when a woman is fearful that the very utterance of her scary thought might startle the therapist or elicit an urgent overreaction. When the therapist responds with a compassionate restatement of the scary thought, although it might still feel unsettling to the woman, the message that she is being heard and cared for is clear.

Fundamentally, the practice of supportive psychotherapy involves the interface between two clinical directives: (a) interventions on behalf of the client, and (b) being with or *holding* the client (Kleiman, 2008; Viederman, 2008; Winnicott, 1987). In this context, holding refers to creating an environment that affords the client the respect and security she needs in order for her to feel safe and cared for. The objective of supportive therapy involves the therapist's attempts to intervene with the preceding goals in mind, such as maximizing adaptive functioning, boosting self-esteem, developing coping strategies, setting appropriate boundaries, minimizing symptoms, and restoring ego strength (Viederman, 2008). *Ego strength* refers to a client's capacity to understand who she is, understand what her capabilities are, and preserve this positive sense of self, despite psychological distress or environmental stressors.

The second and perhaps most central function of supportive psychotherapy involves empathy and the connection between the therapist and the client. Empathy rests between the emotion expressed and the development of the therapeutic relationship. In *Therapy and the Postpartum Woman* (Kleiman, 2008), Karen described the role of the postpartum therapist who uses supportive psychotherapy:

> Within a framework of mutual respect and unconditional acceptance, we listen, we watch, and we care for each client. Not unlike holding the infant with primal needs and impulses, we stay attuned to the new mother's most primitive emotions, what is scaring her, what is immobilizing her, and what is so deep that she can't even put it into words. When we hold on to and tolerate these emotions, managing them without judgment, and without feeling as overwhelmed as she does, we can succeed in containing them. In doing so, we effectively care for her, which is a prerequisite for postpartum healing. (Kleiman, 2008, p. 42)

The clinical model that is followed at The Postpartum Stress Center is delineated in the *voice of depression response model* (Kleiman, 2008). Although this model is geared toward the treating therapist, you may find it validating to learn that the troubling emotions you are experiencing, in conjunction with your scary thoughts, are common and respond well to appropriate support and intervention.

Figure 9.1 illustrates the three primary emotional states that characterize the preponderance of postpartum women in distress: (a) helplessness, (b) fear/anxiety, and/or (c) dependency. The therapist then counters these fragile emotional states with the associated therapeutic responses of reassurance, control, and nurturance. To paraphrase, the therapist offers reassurance to the woman feeling helpless, a sense of control for the woman who experiences uncontrollable anxiety, and nurturance for the woman who feels weakened by her unfamiliar or awkward dependence on others.

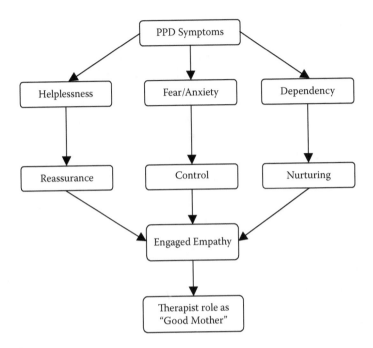

FIGURE 9.1
PPSC Voice of Depression Response Model. (© The Postpartum Stress Center)

When therapists respond with unconditional acceptance to these primary and raw emotional states, they assume the role of the *good mother*. In doing so, they respond in ways that parallel a devoted, tolerant, caring maternal figure, whether the therapist is male or female. When this happens, it enables a postpartum woman to express some of her most urgent needs within a safe setting, paving the way toward empathy, which is a precondition to the success of supportive psychotherapy.

Let's take a closer look at this interaction. The pervasive fear that you will *always feel like this,* or that *this must be how bad a mother is supposed to feel,* or that, perhaps worst of all, *you will never feel better* can accelerate your anxiety considerably. Paying particular attention to the emotional state of anxiety in this model, the supportive therapist's response to your overwhelming anxiety is to acknowledge it and exhibit a sense of *control.* Because the magnitude of anxiety can range from doubting your competency as a mother to the terror that you could injure your baby, feeling out of control can be a gross understatement. When scary thoughts make you feel helpless, fearful, and dependent on others to help sort out genuine concerns from superfluous worry, you may feel both resistant to and desperate for a therapist to offer some perspective.

In response, the role of the supportive therapist is to communicate the conviction that she or he understands the nature of the presenting problem and knows precisely what to do to help you feel better. This point of clarification can offer immediate relief. Sometimes, if you are terrified by your thoughts, this may provide your first glimmer of hope. The therapeutic response of taking control by providing structure, support, guidance, and reassurance serves to model the control you seek in your life. Thus, a woman experiencing scary thoughts can surrender her wish for control, temporarily, by allowing the therapist to take the lead with the hope of obtaining symptom relief. This collaboration is the first step toward *engaged empathy*—the heart of supportive psychotherapy.

By establishing an empathic connection and a sense of security, the supportive therapist can help you overcome feelings of intense anxiety. If you decide to find a supportive psychotherapist, you should expect the following in your sessions (Lipsitz et al., 2008):

- A relaxed conversational style
- A therapist who communicates interest and caring through verbal and nonverbal cues
- Active help with decision making
- Assistance with the expression of emotion
- Praise, encouragement, and reassurance when appropriate
- Empathic statements that help you feel listened to and understood

When these conditions are present, women can expect relief from their intense anxiety and, subsequently, greater command of their scary thoughts.

Cognitive Behavioral Therapy

Cognitive behavioral therapy (CBT) is a short-term, active approach to treatment that assumes a problem-solving focus. The client and therapist collaborate to set treatment goals and to work actively toward meeting them. Clients are usually encouraged to complete assignments outside the sessions. This "homework" is done to ensure that the strategies for managing scary thoughts and emotions addressed in session can be applied in a person's real life outside sessions. CBT was originally developed as a treatment for depression (Beck, Rush, Shaw, & Emery, 1979), and over the past 30 years, it has been applied to a large range of psychiatric problems, especially the ones described in this book.

Most clients who participate in CBT learn strategies to manage their distressing or unhelpful thoughts and emotions. These strategies usually fall into one of two categories: those that are cognitive in nature and those that are behavioral in nature. You already learned about the cognitive strategies in Chapter 8. Cognitive behavioral therapists will use those strategies to help you identify instances when scary thoughts arise and then evaluate them in a systematic manner and draw a more balanced conclusion.

With some practice, clients are able to call upon these strategies as soon as a scary thought comes to mind; in this way, they are able to neutralize the thought before it wreaks emotional havoc. As stated in Chapter 8, over the course of CBT, clients begin to realize that their scary thoughts stem from *core beliefs,* which are deep, fundamental beliefs that one holds about oneself, the world, or the future. Most lasting change comes about when unhelpful beliefs are acknowledged and softened over time.

The cognitive strategies are just one side of the coin. Cognitive behavioral therapists also work with clients to target maladaptive behaviors that cause life interference. One common behavioral strategy is *exposure,* which is systematic confrontation with a feared object, situation, or even a thought or memory. For example, mothers with obsessive thoughts might avoid their babies for fear that they will do something to hurt them, and mothers with intrusive memories might avoid their babies because the baby is a reminder of a traumatic childbirth. A cognitive behavioral therapist encourages these mothers to spend increasingly larger amounts of time with their babies in order to decrease the anxiety.

You might wonder how being in contact with the very thing that is distressing would be therapeutic. Although your anxiety and discomfort are expected to increase when you first go through an exposure exercise, over time, your anxiety will decrease by a process called *habituation* (Wiegartz & Gyoerkoe, 2009). This means that your mind and body adjust to the source of the anxiety, and the initial arousal eventually decreases. Moreover, exposure has beneficial cognitive effects as well, in that it demonstrates that the feared outcomes do not come true.

A related set of behavioral strategies that cognitive behavioral therapists often use with exposure is called *response prevention.* Although it may seem hard to do, this refers to making a choice *not* to act on a compulsive behavior when contacting the very thing that makes you anxious. When mothers have scary thoughts, they often develop elaborate behavioral and avoidance rituals to cope with the anxiety. Examples of these rituals include checking on the baby several times, seeking constant reassurance from a spouse or partner, and engaging in superstitious behavior. However, engaging in these rituals can prevent women from habituating the anxiety. Thus, response prevention helps maximize the benefit of the exposure so that habituation can occur and lead to lasting reductions in scary thoughts and distressing emotions.

Cognitive behavioral therapists also use a number of other behavioral strategies, depending on a client's presenting problem. For example, some people who engage in excessive worry believe that they don't have the skills to solve the problems that they face (Dugas, Gagnon, Ladouceur, & Freeston, 1998). In such a case, the therapist may help the client to acquire adaptive problem-solving skills. Others who are depressed and who ruminate often say they are just going through the motions, getting little enjoyment, pleasure, or meaning from their daily activities. In these cases, cognitive behavioral therapists may work with them to plan pleasurable and meaningful activities in order to increase their engagement with positive aspects of their environment, thereby improving their mood.

This is just a brief overview of a few common strategies used to address scary thoughts and distressing emotions in CBT. An individualized treatment plan will be developed collaboratively between you and your therapist on the basis of the scary thoughts and emotions that are most prominent for you, the ways in which you cope with the thoughts and emotions, your current life circumstances, and your history of psychological distress. You will have the opportunity to provide feedback throughout the course of treatment, so any strategies that you do not view as a good match for your symptoms or life situation will be addressed.

No research has evaluated the effectiveness of CBT for scary thoughts, per se, in postpartum women; however, researchers have evaluated the effectiveness of CBT for some of the postpartum psychiatric disorders described in this book. CBT seems to be as effective as medications and supportive psychotherapy for postpartum depression (Dennis, 2004) and general symptoms of postpartum anxiety (Wenzel, 2011). Although these findings suggest that CBT is a solid treatment option for depressed and anxious postpartum women, it is important to note that the evidence supporting its effectiveness is not as strong as its effectiveness in other populations, in which CBT is often more effective than medications and supportive psychotherapy (Butler, Chapman, Forman, & Beck, 2006).

Part of the reason for this discrepancy is probably that there are procedural limitations to most of the studies that have evaluated CBT in postpartum women (Dennis, 2004). However, it could also be that postpartum women, who are juggling the demands of an infant, find it difficult to implement some of the CBT strategies, which require systematic practice in between sessions. If you found yourself responding well to the strategies described in Chapter 8, then CBT might be a good match for you. Conversely, if you find yourself drawn to one of the other approaches described in this chapter, we would encourage you to pursue that type of treatment.

Interpersonal Psychotherapy

Interpersonal psychotherapy (IPT) is a short-term psychotherapy that focuses on problems in interpersonal relationships and their association with mood disturbance (Weissman, Markowitz, & Klerman, 2000). The therapist and client work actively and collaboratively to identify problematic patterns in current relationships, process emotion associated with those patterns, and change unhelpful expectations, communication styles, or other relationship behaviors. Therapeutic work often falls into one of four interpersonal problem areas: (a) grief, (b) role disputes, (c) role transitions, or (d) interpersonal deficits.

Most postpartum women who participate in IPT focus mainly on the role transition of becoming a parent and any disputes or conflicts that occur during adjustment to this new role. On the surface, CBT might seem like a better match for treating a mother who experiences scary thoughts because a major target of CBT is to modify unhelpful thoughts and beliefs. However, many postpartum women find that IPT is a natural fit for the challenges that they experience during the transition to parenthood.

There is ample evidence that IPT is an effective treatment for postpartum depression. Not only do most women experience a reduction in depressive symptoms, but they also report an improvement in functioning and satisfaction with the partner relationship (O'Hara, Stuart, Gorman, & Wenzel, 2000). Preliminary research raises the possibility that IPT is an effective treatment for panic disorder (Lipsitz et al., 2006) and PTSD (Bleiberg & Markowitz, 2005).

However, IPT has not been evaluated in samples of postpartum women with these anxiety disorders, nor has it been evaluated for GAD and OCD. In addition, no research has been conducted specifically to examine the degree to which IPT is effective in reducing excessive worry, rumination, obsessive thoughts, intrusive memories, and catastrophic misinterpretations of bodily symptoms. IPT might be a good fit for women whose scary thoughts have an interpersonal basis or who are experiencing conflict with others as a result of their scary thoughts.

Group Psychotherapy

Group psychotherapy is another way to integrate the principles of supportive psychotherapy, CBT, and IPT. Sometimes it can be difficult to discern the difference between support groups (described in Chapter 7) and group psychotherapy. Both interventions seek to alleviate the upsetting symptoms of anxiety and depression. Support groups are focused on just what the name implies—providing support. In many instances, support groups are psychoeducational in nature, meaning that attendees learn information about the nature and course of symptoms that they are experiencing. Although many women find that group psychotherapy is also supportive and a place to be educated about their symptoms, they often achieve additional benefits, such as the development and practice of strategies to manage their symptoms and develop new skills. Unlike some support groups, group psychotherapy is always led by a mental health professional.

CBT and IPT, two modes of therapy that have been adapted to the individual treatment of postpartum women, can also be conducted in a group psychotherapy setting. In fact, most of the research on group psychotherapy for postpartum distress evaluates one of these two modalities. This research shows that group CBT and group IPT are associated with reductions in depressive and anxious symptoms from pretreatment to posttreatment and that they are usually more effective in doing so than the care that women typically would receive if their healthcare provider recognized that they needed treatment for postpartum distress (Wenzel, 2011).

To our knowledge, research has not yet been conducted to compare the effectiveness of individual or group psychotherapy for postpartum distress. Such research has been conducted with those seeking treatment for depression or anxiety, and it generally shows no difference between modalities in their effectiveness (e.g., Lockwood, Page, & Connor-Hiller, 2004). However, once again, we need to emphasize that no research has specifically investigated the manner in which scary thoughts change as a result of participation in group psychotherapy.

How do you choose between individual and group psychotherapy? One notion is simply to pay close attention to your preferences: Would you prefer the undivided attention of a therapist or would you prefer to work with other women who are going through similar issues? You might also consider the number and extent of symptoms, life problems, and issues that you'd like to address in psychotherapy. By and large, group psychotherapy will only target the symptoms or issues that are the topic of the group, such as "postpartum adjustment." In contrast, you might start out by addressing postpartum adjustment issues in individual psychotherapy, but you might also want to work on other unrelated or longer standing issues. In the latter case, individual psychotherapy could be a wise choice because a therapeutic relationship with a trusted healthcare provider would be in place as you address the unrelated or longer standing issues. Finally, your choice might be driven, in part, by practical considerations. If you'd like to work with a professional therapist but no therapy groups are available in your locale, then individual psychotherapy might be the best option. In some cases, women use both.

MEDICATIONS

Another option for treatment of postpartum distress is to take one or more *psychotropic medications,* which are defined as medications that target psychiatric or emotional symptoms. Although we are sensitive to the fact that many postpartum women are reluctant to consider taking these medications, it is important that you have all the information in front of you so that you can be the best advocate for your healthcare decisions.

Psychotropic medications (e.g., antidepressants or antianxiety medications) are prescribed by a medical doctor, such as your obstetrician, primary doctor, a psychiatrist, or, under the supervision of a medical doctor, a nurse practitioner or physician's assistant. Oftentimes, you will be started on a relatively low dosage of a medication and instructed to schedule a follow-up appointment within a designated short period of time (e.g., 4 weeks).

Then, at the time of the next visit, depending on your symptoms, a decision is made whether or not to increase your dosage. Although medication management by one of these healthcare professionals requires in-person visits, they are usually less frequent than visits for psychotherapy, and they often last for a shorter period of time (e.g., 15–30 minutes for a medication check vs. 50–60 minutes for an individual psychotherapy session). Antidepressants typically take several weeks to effect positive changes.

Many postpartum women, understandably, have significant concerns about taking medications while they are breastfeeding. At present, although no guidelines have been published by the Food and Drug Administration (FDA) for the use of these medications in lactating women, though we expect that the FDA will do so within the next few years. For now, healthcare providers make recommendations about the use of psychotropic medications on the basis of (a) research that has documented effects of these medications in breastfeeding infants, and (b) mothers' preferences. All of the medications described in this section have either no evidence that their use is associated with adverse effects in the infant or evidence of only minimal, non-life-threatening effects (Hale, 2008). Even so, if you are not comfortable taking one of these medications while you are nursing, you should discuss this with your doctor and consider some of the other interventions described in this chapter.

Antidepressants

Although the name *antidepressant* suggests that these medications target depression, they are used just as frequently to treat anxiety. Thus, antidepressants would be a reasonable choice of intervention to treat any one of the types of scary thoughts described in this book and the distress that they cause. The most commonly prescribed category of antidepressants is the serotonin reuptake inhibitors, of which there are two types: (a) selective serotonin reuptake inhibitors (SSRIs), and (b) serotonin-norepinephrine reuptake inhibitors (SNRIs). Serotonin and norepinephrine are neurotransmitters that are involved in the regulation of mood. Serotonin reuptake inhibitors work by "recycling" the targeted neurotransmitters and allowing more time for them to do their jobs.

Commonly prescribed SSRIs include citalopram (Celexa), escitalopram (Lexapro), fluoxetine (Prozac), fluvoxamine (Luvox), paroxetine (Paxil), and sertraline (Zoloft). Commonly prescribed SNRIs include duloxetine

(Cymbalta) and venlafaxine (Effexor). Desvenlafaxine (Pristiq) is another SNRI that has been recently introduced on the market. It is a metabolite of venlafaxine, which means that the research on venlafaxine should apply; however, at the time we are writing this book, no research is available on the effects of this medication on the nursing infant.

Typical side effects of these medications include loss of appetite, sleep disturbance, headaches, fatigue, nausea, urinary retention, and sexual dysfunction (i.e., loss of interest, difficulty achieving orgasm). Although this list of side effects may seem daunting, keep in mind that most people only experience a subset of these side effects, and the side effects often subside after a few weeks of use.

Postpartum women who are breastfeeding are typically less interested in the side effects that *they* experience from serotonin reuptake inhibitors and more interested in effects on their nursing babies. Excretion of these medications into the breast milk is relatively low, so the infant is only exposed to a small amount of the medication (Eberhard-Gran, Eskild, & Opjordsmoen, 2006). In fact, one group of experts (Ragan, Stowe, & Newport, 2005) stated that a child would have to breastfeed for over 2 years to get the same exposure to medication that occurs during only 1 month of pregnancy.

Adverse effects that have been observed in infants are mainly limited to colic, gastrointestinal problems, and sleep disturbance (Eberhard-Gran et al., 2006; Ragan et al., 2005). There can also be short-lived withdrawal symptoms of a similar nature when infants are weaned from breastfeeding mothers who take serotonin reuptake inhibitors (Kristensen et al., 1999). It is often recommended that the best serotonin reuptake inhibitors to prescribe are those that are metabolized by the mother in a relatively short time. It is also possible for a nursing mother to "pump and dump." This technique consists of pumping and then disposing of the breast milk at the time when the medication would be deemed most prominent in the milk, thereby reducing the infant's exposure.

Your healthcare provider may consider other types of antidepressants. Bupropion (Wellbutrin) is regarded as an atypical antidepressant that inhibits the reuptake of norepinephrine and dopamine, allowing these neurotransmitters more time to exert action. Side effects include seizures (rare), agitation, and sleep disturbance. Although case studies show that bupropion is generally undetected in mothers' milk or in infant plasma levels, one case study documented seizures in an infant whose mother took this medication (Hale, 2008). It also is important to consider that although current data support the use of Bupropion for depression, similar research has not been conducted for the anxiety disorders described in this book.

Tricyclic antidepressants are older antidepressants that inhibit the reuptake of three neurotransmitters: serotonin, norepinephrine, and dopamine. Examples of medications in this class are imipramine (Tofranil) and clomipramine (Anafranil). People who take tricyclic antidepressants tend to experience more side effects than do people who take serotonin reuptake inhibitors; these include dry mouth, blurry vision, constipation, and urinary retention. For this reason, tricyclic antidepressants usually are not the first drugs prescribed for people with anxiety and depression, unless they have had positive responses to these medications in the past. The sparse research that has been conducted on tricyclic antidepressant use while breastfeeding suggests few, if any, adverse side effects on nursing infants.

Finally, monoamine oxidase inhibitors (MAOIs) are antidepressants that work by preventing the breakdown of neurotransmitters such as serotonin and norepinephrine by inhibiting an enzyme called monoamine oxidase. However, these medications are rarely the first medication of choice because their use requires significant dietary restrictions, and there is the potential for dangerous interactions with other drugs. Moreover, the effects of MAOIs on nursing infants have not been examined in the literature, so their use in lactating women should be undertaken with extreme caution.

Evidence for the efficacy of antidepressants in treating anxiety and depression in postpartum women is limited to case studies; in fact, the body of research on psychotherapy for postpartum distress is better developed than the body of research on antidepressants for treating postpartum distress. However, there is much evidence for the efficacy of antidepressants for reducing symptoms associated with anxiety and depression in the general population (e.g., Papakostas, Thase, Fava, Nelson, & Shelton, 2007). If you and your healthcare professional decide that antidepressants would be right for you, you will work together to find the medication that best meets your needs. Keep in mind that sometimes this is a "trial-and-error" process and some women need to try several antidepressants before finding the one that works best for them.

Antianxiety Agents

Antianxiety agents are typically prescribed for acute anxiety and, in some instances, for sleep disturbance. Two types of antianxiety agents are prescribed for the anxiety associated with scary thoughts: benzodiazepines and buspirone. Benzodiazepines, or minor tranquilizers, exert their action on a neurotransmitter called gamma-amniobutyric acid (GABA). Examples of benzopdiazepines include alprazolam (Xanax), clonazepam (Klonopin), diazepam (Valium), and lorazepam (Ativan). Unlike antidepressant medications, benzopdiazepines work very quickly, and many people notice their effects within a half hour to an hour of taking the medication. For this reason, healthcare providers may prescribe these medications on an as-needed basis so that women can take them only in instances in which their anxiety is acute.

Women who take benzodiazepines experience a different group of side effects than they experience with antidepressants, most noticeably drowsiness and, rarely, short-term cognitive or memory impairment. Prolonged use may be associated with the development of tolerance and dependence, and women may experience withdrawal symptoms when they discontinue using them. For these reasons, antidepressants are often the first medication considered to treat anxiety, with antianxiety agents used for relief in the short term until antidepressants take effect.

Most research suggests that only trace amounts of benzodiazepines are found in infant serum levels, although some case studies have documented adverse effects in nursing infants, such as breathing difficulties, lethargy, sedation, and feeding problems (Hale, 2008) associated with high doses or high frequency of taking the medication. If benzodiazepines are indicated for a breastfeeding woman, it is recommended that the fastest acting medication be used, which is more easily metabolized by the baby's liver (e.g., lorazepam); thus, the infant is exposed to the smallest possible amount. Although no research has examined the efficacy of benzodiazepines in treating postpartum distress, research with people who suffer from anxiety suggests that they are effective in treating GAD and panic disorder (Wenzel, 2011).

Buspirone (BuSpar) is an antianxiety agent that exerts its action on serotonin receptors. Unlike benzodiazepines, there is no addictive potential associated with the use of buspirone, although it typically takes up to 4 weeks to notice its effects. Although this safety profile might indicate that buspirone is safer to take than benzodiazepines while breastfeeding, it is prescribed with caution in nursing mothers because research has yet to identify its concentration in breast milk or document effects in nursing infants (Hale, 2008). Data indicate that buspirone is efficacious in treating GAD, but as we have seen with the other medications described in this section, no research has examined the efficacy of buspirone in the treatment of postpartum distress.

GOING FORWARD WITH TREATMENT

It has been suggested that possibly the most significant relief from anxiety arises from the action taken to engage in some treatment intervention, regardless of what that treatment actually is (Milgrom, Negri, Gemmill, McNeil, & Martin, 2005). Thus, if you are frightened by your thoughts and decide to seek professional help, the specific modality you choose is less important than the fact that you are getting help. The bottom line here is that the decision process regarding whether or not to pursue a particular intervention strategy always involves a risk-benefit analysis. What is the risk of not getting help? What is the risk of taking medication? What is the risk of not taking medication?

Sometimes, women perceive the act of getting help as a sign of weakness; they believe they should be strong enough to tackle their anxiety or depression on their own. Another misperception is that the mere act of "doing something" carries greater risk than sitting back and doing nothing. But sometimes not doing anything is associated with tremendous risk (e.g., not going to the doctor when you have chest pains), and the cost of hoping things go away on their own can have devastating ramifications.

Therefore, if you are feeling anxious about the thoughts you are having, the price of doing nothing is high. We have seen that wishing the thoughts away will not work. Weighing the risks and benefits of the professional interventions discussed in this chapter will help you move forward on a course of action that is best suited to you. Some things for you to consider include:

- Has medication been helpful to you in the past?
- Has medication been helpful to family members?

- Are you breastfeeding?
- Do you think you can find the resources to support you during this stressful time?
- Has psychotherapy been helpful to you in the past?
- Do you tend to like structured settings with assignments to guide your work on your areas of vulnerability?
- Do you think your relationships are the key to understanding and addressing your feelings of anxiety and/or depression?
- Do group settings make you feel anxious or are you comforted by the presence of others?
- Do you have supportive, reliable contacts with whom you can discuss treatment options?

The crux of this issue is that you need to make sure you are informed of your options. You need to advocate for your own best healthcare. What may be right for one woman may not be best for you. Your instincts, your preferences, your personal history, and the extent to which you are suffering, along with the input from loved ones and healthcare providers, will combine to lead you in a direction that feels most accommodating and beneficial at this time.

Take-Home Point for Mothers. If you do not like the way you are feeling, you've been feeling bad for a while, you've tried several self-help strategies and nothing is providing enough relief, or you still think something is terribly wrong with you and the way you are thinking, then it's time to seek support from a healthcare professional. Someone who is well-trained in treating pregnant and postpartum women will understand what you are experiencing and know what you need to start to feel better. Do not suffer longer than you already have. If you're not sure whether you really need to see a healthcare professional, call one anyway and let that individual help you sort it out.

Clinician Note. A postpartum woman who has come to you for support and clarification has, most likely, been suffering with acute anxiety for some time. She may even be coming to you after seeing one or more previous healthcare providers or clinicians who have dismissed her feelings or overreacted to them. You are in position to make a significant difference in how she is feeling, almost immediately, by sharing what you know and validating her experience.

10

How Others Can Help

The struggle with anxiety and depression is hard to go through alone. As we've seen, it's also hard to talk about it and reach out for help. Support provided by extended family and healthcare providers protects the physical and psychological health of postpartum women. All forms of support, including economic assistance, practical household help, and emotional encouragement, can ease a mother's stress. In fact, research has shown that mothers who perceive themselves as well supported during pregnancy report minimal symptoms of depression during the postpartum period (O'Hara & Swain, 1996). Because greater social support can reduce anxiety and because scary thoughts are manifestations of anxiety, it follows that social support can minimize the impact of the scary thoughts themselves. It looks like this:

Social support → reduced stress → decreased distress → weakening of scary thoughts

Because support has protective properties against anxiety, it is important to explore the mechanisms that enhance or inhibit the development of a support system. In this way, women can help fortify their resources and better defend themselves against the force of scary thoughts.

WHAT EXACTLY DO WE MEAN BY SUPPORT?

In *This Isn't What I Expected* (Kleiman & Raskin, 1994), Karen outlined two categories of support that are critical for new mothers: practical support and emotional support. *Practical support* is defined as hands-on help or assistance with tasks and includes things that others can do or provide that will lighten the new mother's responsibilities, such as doing laundry, shopping for the family, and babysitting. *Emotional support* involves a relationship that serves to ease the burden through intangible gifts, such as comfort, reassurance, intimacy, validation, and encouragement.

A third category of support is *psychosocial support*, which includes information, programs, or groups that help promote healthy attitudes and skills related to mothering and maternal mental health. Psychosocial support could take the form of support groups, mother's meetings, or other organized forums that have been developed to improve adjustment to this major life transition. Psychosocial support is especially important when a low-income or any at-risk population, which may have limited access to professional resources, is considered. Regardless of a woman's access to help, any kind of support can be difficult to ask for if she is not in the habit of or comfortable in doing so.

Measuring social support involves more than just taking account of a woman's access to personal resources. Think about it. The concept of support itself implies an interaction between environmental or external resources and the woman herself. A woman can be exposed to an abundance of resources, but if she is not inclined to extend herself or take advantage of what is available, the resources will have little value. Thus, social support pertains not only to the resources to which a woman has access, but also to the extent to which she utilizes these resources and finds them helpful.

Asking for Help: What Gets in the Way and Why?

Women tend to take better care of everyone else than they do of themselves. Most women readily confess that self-care is on the bottom of their "to-do" lists. Mothers, in particular, are inclined to sacrifice their own needs while maintaining intense focus on the needs of their children. Often, mothers are motivated by the belief that complete and singular attention to their child is the very hallmark of a devoted, loving mother. Compromise in this area does not feel like an option to many women.

This prevailing notion that motherhood is synonymous with sacrifice—if not complete abandonment—of one's own needs can quickly translate into a loss of self. Somewhere along the way, mothers have incorporated the misperception that taking care of themselves is selfish and incompatible with the fierce demands of motherhood.

It's hard to ask for help. Asking for help is often perceived as a character weakness: *If I were only strong enough, I could do this by myself,* or worse, a mothering flaw: *If I were a good mother, I wouldn't need help.* Giving help is simply easier than asking for it, and accepting it is even harder altogether! However, it is important to recognize that these perceptions are just that—*perceptions*—rather than facts.

In early chapters, we learned that mothers with scary thoughts are understandably reluctant to let others know how they are feeling and what they are thinking. Even though a mother might understand that it is in her best interest to talk about it, it makes sense that she might hesitate to do so. Nevertheless, asking for help around the house, help with the kids, or companionship to ease the strain is essential to a woman's well-being and should surpass the reflex not to ask for it. All of the strategies described in Chapter 8 to address scary thoughts can also be used to address perceptions of inadequacy, character weakness, and flaws in the context of asking for help.

One of the most powerful contributing factors to a woman's reluctance to ask for help during the postpartum period is her need for control when everything around her seems to be so out of control. During this time when unpredictability triumphs over order, postpartum women are often forced to relinquish their desire for harmony and settle for the illusion of control. What does an illusion of control look like? It looks perfect. If a woman is inclined toward perfectionism, this tendency will promptly supersede the chaos. In this way, everything that feels out of place miraculously falls in line. At least that's how it looks. One new mother described it this way:

> I tried so hard to make sure everyone saw me as a mother who was totally in control; after all, I've done this before. No big deal. Women have been having babies for centuries. I knew what I needed to do to look good so no one would think anything was wrong. On the surface, it looked exactly the way I wanted it to. I was calm and perfectly in control. I made sure to put my makeup on right before an appointment with my doctor or my kid's doctor or my therapist. I even put on lipstick, which I never wear, so I would look fresh and ready for the world. But it was like my body was stuck in high idle with my engine revving but going nowhere. At any moment, I felt my insides would rupture. Still, I wouldn't dare let anyone know I was feeling that way.

The energy it takes to maintain this illusion is enormous and, ironically, makes it harder to ask for help. The experience of feeling completely out of control, while simultaneously longing for it, is not unfamiliar to mothers. This is why it is so important for women to give themselves permission to ask for help. Remember that the objective is to reduce the external stress and thereby reduce the distress, and, in so doing, reduce the frequency or intensity of the scary thoughts.

Asking for help is not a luxury. It is essential.

Asking for Help: Now and Now

The concept of asking for help entails one core assumption. It requires a basic belief in the power of meaningful relationships. If someone truly believes that no one or nothing could ever help, there is no reason to ask for anything. But if there is even a spark of hope—the slightest possibility of relief in the not-so-distant future—one is more motivated to summon the courage to ask for assistance in some way. Interpersonal connection is the key to much of the healing that needs to take place during the postpartum period (Kleiman, 2008). When postpartum women feel listened to and cared for, they become more resilient to the onslaught of intense emotions and overwhelming distress.

In order to best utilize the support available to you, you first need to determine with whom you feel most comfortable discussing your feelings. Next, you should assume a proactive posture in regard to what you need. You must resist the temptation to isolate or further withdraw from available resources. Reach out. Call a friend. Talk to your partner. Confide in your healthcare provider. Include your mother, your mother-in-law, your neighbor, or your sister. Find the one person or the two or the many people with whom you feel most safe and then take a leap of faith that they will follow through with the support you need. Consider the following when you are reaching out:

- **Who** (What is your relationship with this person? Who would come to mind if you needed to make a call in the middle of the night?)
- **Timing** (Are other things going on at this time that may prevent this person from helping at this time? If so, is that based in reality, or do you perceive your request to be a burden of sorts?)

- **Why** (What are your expectations? Why do you think this person would make himself or herself available to you?)

Scary thoughts are scary to you and potentially to those around you. We have seen that without proper information, the impact of thoughts that are left to the imagination can swirl out of control, wreaking emotional havoc. In our practices, we have discovered that clients, family members, and healthcare providers all need more information about postpartum anxiety and, in particular, about the specific nature of scary thoughts. When it comes to understanding scary thoughts, it seems that everyone shares an equal disadvantage: It puts almost everyone on edge.

The flip side to asking for help is accepting it when it is offered—and accepting it without guilt. This is an essential part of self-care. Letting others rally around you so that you can heal and continue to feel strong is essential. Once you can find the right people with whom you can share your thoughts, you need to be clear about what reaching out to them means to you and what they need to do (and not do) in response. In other words, let them know this is hard to talk about and why it's so important that they listen.

Getting the Most From Your Support Network

One research study found that the greater number of social support providers to whom a woman was connected, the greater the positive impact on postpartum adjustment (Logsdon, Birkimer, & Barbee, 1997). In other words, the more people a postpartum woman had to turn to for a variety of issues, the more supported she felt. Although that may seem too obvious to mention, it's worth noting in order to reemphasize the value of creating or strengthening an existing network of support. When a support network is maximized, distress is lowered.

This same study demonstrated that postpartum women reported needing help in three areas: (a) day-to-day concerns, (b) ability to carry out activities due to illness, and (c) urgent needs. The authors stated, "Doing household chores, running errands, and caring for others dominate the lives of young mothers; thus they seek help most for these areas, particularly when their physical health is compromised, as it often is after childbirth" (Logsdon et al., 1997, p. 94). These types of practical support can help reduce the stress inundating a new mother.

Conversely, research also shows that *negative social support* (defined as negative interactions with people in one's support network) exacerbates stress and anxiety. Amy's former student found that only negative social support, rather than the number of people in a woman's support network or the woman's satisfaction with her support network, predicted anxiety at 8 weeks postpartum (Haugen, 2003). What this means is that, just as it is important to be mindful and open to the positive support you are receiving, it is also important to recognize when others who mean to be supportive are experienced as intrusive or unhelpful.

Support From Your Friends and Other Moms

One thing is certain: The more you isolate yourself, the more your thoughts will be all consuming. It may very well be what you feel most like doing, but it is almost certain to increase your anxiety and make you feel worse. The mere activity of joining others can create a distraction for your busy brain. And if you're lucky enough to be surrounded by friends who are also new moms, you will likely find that they share many of your anxieties. In addition to the types of support groups mentioned in Chapter 7, there are new mother groups that offer classes, play groups, monthly meetings, or casual get-togethers for moms and their children. Participation in these structured groups may help to normalize your thoughts, either by discussing them or getting information to help refute them.

Relationship With Your Partner

When acute distress sets in, women who suffer don't typically rush to understand the particular brain dysregulation or the biological mechanisms that underlie these bizarre thinking patterns. Instead, they might panic, shut down, or search for immediate help. By far, partners topped the list of those people to whom women initially disclose their feelings of anxiety and of being overwhelmed during the postpartum period. Our experience has shown that regardless of the perceived level of support or strength of the marital bond, women almost automatically express concern about their high levels of anxiety to their partners when they are scared by how they are feeling.

When a partner's reaction is sympathetic, it is followed by much needed respite from the heartache. Such a response can go a long way to ease the burden if there is an expression of trust, reassurance, and confidence that everything will be okay (Kleiman, 2000). Conversely, if a partner's reaction is unhelpful, patronizing, or dismissive, these attempts to reach out might be stuffed away or shut down. This is why it is essential that partners are informed and understand the unique nature of scary thoughts.

Remember Jen from Chapter 7, who was unfamiliar with intense anxiety until the birth of her second child? She became afraid that her husband wouldn't be able to handle her anxiety because she had always been a pillar of strength within the family system. She described herself as the go-to person for everyone. She was the one her sisters and her friends ran to whenever they needed anything. She feared all would crumble if she admitted the extent to which she felt immobilized by her scary thoughts and images. She described her reluctance to let her husband know how she was feeling:

> I was so certain Jon would totally freak out if I told him I had thoughts of our baby dying. Especially when I was thinking that I could hurt her with our knives or his hammer or the car. It was completely unnerving. I thought for sure he would leave me or tell me I was nuts. He's so used to me being in control. I thought either he wouldn't take me seriously or he would totally go ballistic. Worrying about telling him was almost as painful as the thoughts themselves. When my therapist told me she believed Jon would be able to tolerate it and that it might help me feel better, I decided I had no choice but to talk to him. When you feel bad enough, something kicks in, I guess; it becomes a matter of survival.

Jen ultimately discovered that the strength of her relationship was able to sustain the exposure of her thoughts and images. Moreover, it was helpful when she brought Jon to her therapy session so that he could get more information and become more comfortable with the situation. Here, again, we see how the grip of anxiety can obscure thinking and make it difficult to trust one's instincts. It's hard to find clarity and make sense out of things when thoughts are cluttered by distortion or symptoms. For this reason, it is even more crucial for women to let someone know when they are struggling. The objectivity of another's perspective can help clarify some of the confusion.

Unfortunately, sometimes disclosing the nature of scary thoughts to a partner backfires. It can be devastating to make oneself vulnerable and reach out only to feel smacked by some unconstructive response. A partner might respond insufficiently because of his own denial, anxiety, or panic. Or, a dismissive response might reflect his lack of understanding, leading to impatience, irritability, or mockery. If this happens to you, try not to let this be too discouraging. Remember that it is scary for him too. He needs the right information so that he can be onboard and help you feel supported. It may not make sense, but sometimes it's worth it to do the extra work in order to help him help you. The payoff can be significant.

Good communication and conflict resolution skills are associated with high-functioning marriages (Papp, Goeke-Morey, & Cummings, 2007), so it is essential that partners not lose sight of that, even when anxiety is at its peak. Open, honest discussions and strategies that perpetuate them are mechanisms that inspire thriving marriages. Talk whether you feel like it or not. Reach out for support whether or not you view yourself worthy or competent to ask for it. Many postpartum women continue to suffer in silence for fear of "rocking the boat"—asking for too much or starting a fight or disappointing their partner. Learning how to problem solve is a key ingredient to the well-being of your marriage. Resist the temptation to shy away from this. It will make things feel better, or it will reveal areas of vulnerability in your relationship that could use some attention and reinforcement.

MESSAGE TO FAMILY MEMBERS AND OTHER SUPPORT PERSONS

If you are trying to understand and support a loved one who is struggling with scary thoughts, it can feel overwhelming and frightening. How do you know if her thoughts will lead to action? How do you know if her thoughts are an indication of a serious mental health concern that requires immediate and aggressive intervention? Undoubtedly, her scary thoughts will stir up your own anxiety, as you wonder what the best plan of action at this time would be.

The Postpartum Stress Center created an assessment guide for healthcare providers that has also proven to be helpful for family members. The content of this card reviews much of what has appeared throughout this book. This review of the salient points can help defray anxiety by clarifying what is really going on.

Ways in Which to Provide Support

The most important thing you can do for someone you love who is struggling with scary thoughts is to let her know you understand that this is common, you are not scared by this, and you will be there for her. Scary thoughts make it difficult to ask for help. Offer it. Do your best to learn more about this so that you can better understand the impact this phenomenon can have on her life. Understand that fear can be paralyzing.

WHAT ARE SCARY THOUGHTS?

- Scary thoughts are a very common symptom of postpartum depression and anxiety.
- Scary thoughts are defined as negative, repetitive, unwanted, or intrusive thoughts that can bombard a woman, who feels as if they come out of nowhere.
- The majority of mothers (91%) and fathers (88%) report intrusive thoughts about their baby at some point following the baby's birth (Abramowitz, Khandker, Nelson, Deacon, & Rygwall, 2006).
- Scary thoughts can come in the form of thoughts (*What if I burn the baby in the bath?*), images (visions of the baby falling down the stairs), or impulses (*What if I can't help it and I hurt my baby?*). Scary thoughts can be indirect or passive (*Something might happen to the baby*) or they can imply intention.
- Scary thoughts are NOT an indication of psychosis. They can make a woman feel as if she is going crazy, but she is not.
- **A mother's anxiety or distress over these thoughts is a good sign.** This means the thoughts are anxiety driven and will respond well to treatment.
- Scary thoughts can be part of a general anxiety or mood disorder, or they may occur in the absence of this diagnosis.
- Women who disclose that they are having scary thoughts and report distress and life interference should be referred to a mental health provider who can assess for proper treatment.

(© The Postpartum Stress Center).

Your reassurance and support can provide incredible nourishment when she feels so fragile. Sit with her. Listen to her. Reassure her. If she has expressed concern that she is unable to manage her scary thoughts, ask her if she would feel better if she got professional help; then, assist her with that process. Remind her that there is no shame in asking for help. It takes great courage and strength of character to say, *I don't like the way I am feeling. I am ready to ask someone to help me feel better.* Help her do that.

As you continue to provide support, it will be helpful to follow the guidelines in the following subsections.

Trust Your Instincts

This is the same truism we profess to postpartum women who are suffering. If you think something is wrong, you are probably right. This does not mean that anything terrible is happening. It means that your intuition is sending out a distress signal, and the best response to that is to honor it, take it seriously, and seek support. It also means that everyone will feel better if more information is obtained and all bases are covered. It is prudent to have a professional assess the situation if everyone involved is worried, in the unlikely event that other variables are contributing to her suffering.

Listen to What She Is Telling You

This is not always easy because it may require your setting aside your own anxiety to hear what she is trying to tell you. Ask her what she is afraid of. Try to tolerate her anxiety. Remember that anxiety will not hurt her; it will just feel terrible to her. Remind her that she is safe and that you will be okay no matter what she wants to share. If you do not feel you are able to endure this level of anxiety, be honest about that with yourself and with her, and find someone to help you help her.

Avoid Empty Words of Cheer

Remember that sweeping reassurances when you are not confident about the nature of her suffering may not be helpful. Telling her that everything will be fine when you are not clear how much she is suffering or saying you know how she feels when you do not will not help. Rather, you should validate how bad this must feel to her. Find the balance between taking her seriously and not appearing startled.

Confront Gently

Here is a sequential guide for initiating a dialogue if you are worried about a loved one; it captures many of the points included in this section:

- Ask her if she is having thoughts that are scaring her.
- Ask her what you can do to help.
- Ask her whether she would feel better if she talked to you about the specifics.
- Gently review for her what you have learned about anxiety and the nature of scary thoughts in general in order to restore her confidence that you can handle this.
- Ask her if she thinks she can manage the thoughts or if she would feel better finding a therapist or doctor who can help her.
- State clearly that you believe her if she says she is not going to hurt the baby or act on any of the thoughts that might be scaring her.

Remember that your greatest act of support will be your absolute acceptance of how she is feeling and what she may tell you. Your ability to be present with her in spite of her remorse and self-condemnation will help heal her broken spirit. Never underestimate the meaning and value of truly unconditional support.

The following list is a summary of the decisive points for you to keep in mind:

- Scary thoughts are extremely common; almost all postpartum women have them.
- Even though they are common, they can also be disabling.
- Scary thoughts do not lead to action, although women fear that they will.
- Scary thoughts are associated with anxiety and are not a sign of psychosis, although they can make a woman feel and fear that she is going crazy.

- It may be painful for you to witness her fear, but her fear of her thoughts is actually a good sign. Her fear indicates that the scary thoughts are a symptom of intense anxiety that can be managed or treated professionally.

Warning Signs That Professional Intervention Is Needed

First and foremost, any time you are worried about a loved one who is suffering, it is time to seek professional support. Sometimes it is difficult to determine if more help is needed because she may be hiding how she is feeling or what she is thinking. Additionally, you may overreact or under-react to some of what you see or hear because she is on an emotional roller coaster right now. Keep in mind that the postpartum period is a time of dramatic fluctuation regarding feelings and responses. Senses are heightened, and anxiety is at an all-time high. For this reason, it's hard for her, and it's hard on you to establish whether or not what she is feeling is okay.

If, at any time, you hear concern about her ability to get through the day, her functioning is severely impaired, or she reveals that she feels everyone would be better off without her here, it is time for immediate support. Keep in mind that even passive thoughts of "not being here" constitute suicidal thoughts. Examples of these kinds of statements are *I wish I could just go to sleep and not wake up; I don't want to kill myself but I wish I weren't here; My baby would be better off with another mother.* All of these statements are indications that the risk of suicidal behavior is increased; this requires professional intervention.

A Word to Therapists Who Treat Postpartum Women: Intervention Strategies

When distress is high, postpartum women often experience an alarming disconnect from themselves and from others around them. The self-absorbing preoccupation with how they feel makes it seem impossible to engage in meaningful ways. Women become excessively self-conscious and may feel that everyone around them is moving forward, leaving them wedged between where they are and where they want to be. As with all psychotherapy, the most immediate clinical intervention hinges on the relationship. Similar to a loved one who must convey a sense of control and lack of fear, the therapeutic relationship can do much to inspire a sense of well-being. Connecting to this process is essential for a woman in distress.

Keep these clinical guidelines in mind in order to maximize a woman's connection to the therapeutic process:

1. Be aware of your own areas of strength and vulnerability regarding the expression and treatment of scary thoughts. Seek consultation or supervision when needed. It may or may not surprise you to hear that there are a fairly large number of therapists who express concern about their ability to respond appropriately to the admission of scary thoughts. In her postgraduate training program, Karen reminds ongoing groups of therapists that taking care of their personal and emotional vulnerability is paramount when working with this population. Some therapists, especially novice ones, wonder if they will feel shocked by a thought revealed or an image described in graphic detail. Therapists need to make certain they are fully informed and comfortable differentiating what requires clarification and reassurance from that which should be referred for further psychiatric support.

2. Be clear about your expertise in this area so that there is no room for ambivalence or second guessing. In *Therapy and the Postpartum Woman,* Karen brings to light one of a therapist's greatest challenges:

> Perhaps our greatest resource to promote healing that comes from within us is presented in seemingly contradictory terms. We are, indeed, experts who know nothing. Each woman brings to us her own history, struggle, perspective and resources. We must project authority on this subject yet remain open to that which our clients reveal to and need from us. As we listen with an impartial ear, we set aside our emotional reactivity and desire for a quick fix and return to a state of calm presence. We must simply be there. (Kleiman, 2008, pp. 279–280)

Therapists who work with postpartum women need to know that scary thoughts are a probable part of postpartum clinical work and must be addressed directly. With empathy, this follows as a natural course of the therapeutic alliance. Without empathy, it will lead you both astray.

3. Be firm about your ability to help her. We've seen how difficult it can be for a postpartum woman to ask for help. Once she does, it is imperative that therapists respond with unwavering confidence in their ability to provide that help or facilitate contact with those that can.

4. State and restate what scary thoughts are, what they mean, and what they do not mean. It will likely be beneficial for therapists to reiterate what they know to be true about the nature of scary thoughts so that the client hears it again and again. Equally important is the therapist's demeanor. The client may expect her words to shock an unsuspecting therapist, so it is crucial that the response remain neutral. Body language, facial expression, posture, and spoken words should all signify calm, nonjudgmental feedback.

5. Let her know that she is likely to feel better if she talks about her scary thoughts. Remind the client that she is safe and that the amount of energy it takes to hold tight to the shame and pain of a secret can be grueling. There can be great satisfaction in sharing the burden with someone she trusts. When the relationship develops successfully and enables the emergence of empathy, this disclosure of scary thoughts becomes a more natural outcome.

Take-Home Point for Mothers. One of your greatest resources right now is your access to support from people who care about you. Identify it, access it, and rely on it. There is great restorative and healing power within the relationships that are most meaningful to you. Do not let feelings of uncertainty, embarrassment, or guilt deny you from getting the support you need and deserve.

Clinician Note. You may hold the key to unlocking a postpartum woman from the prison of her scary thoughts. Your commitment to her well-being and your precise knowledge of what is happening (and what is *not* happening) will provide initial and enduring hopefulness. This hopefulness, as we know, translates into motivation and dedication to the healing process.

11

Your Personal Treatment Plan

We anticipate that, at this point, you are feeling more informed and, hopefully, slightly less anxious about some of the thoughts you are having. What will help now (though it might temporarily increase your anxiety a bit) is an honest assessment of what you are experiencing in order to break the cycle of scary thoughts and restore a sense of emotional equilibrium. An authentic appraisal, as such, includes the recognition and acceptance of the anxiety that may continue to stream through your mind, infecting your perceptions. That is, your desire for the distress to disappear completely is unrealistic, regardless of the work you do or the help that you receive. Our hope for you is that by reading this book and following some of our suggestions, you will effectively be able to decrease your anxiety, learn to manage that which remains, and come to peace with who you are, with or without distress.

This chapter is designed to gather the material we have described up to this point and propose a recovery plan that is exclusively yours. This will enable you to think through what you are experiencing and put a name to it, which should curtail your feelings of isolation and shame. Tackling your scary thoughts at close range is not easy. Your intention to follow through and your determination to lessen your suffering should motivate you throughout this process. As you work through this chapter, you may want to refer back to the earlier chapters for details about the nature and origins of scary thoughts, as well as specific strategies that can help you to manage them.

There are eight steps to break the scary-thought cycle. Although these steps have been referenced throughout this book, they now serve as a guide to better understand your unique situation and determine the best course of action. As you proceed through these stages, the workbook format will enable you to record your specific concerns and develop a plan of action that is best suited to you and what you need.

BREAKING THE CYCLE: EIGHT STEPS

- Acknowledgment
- Identification
- Disclosure and barriers
- Vulnerabilities
- Self-help and nonprofessional interventions
- Cognitive strategies
- Professional treatment options
- Acceptance

Acknowledgment

You are having scary thoughts. Acknowledging that something as upsetting as this exists does not mean you have to like it. Nor does it mean you have completely accepted the thoughts' reason for being. Those are steps you will tackle later, perhaps after you have absorbed what you have learned. For now, we ask that you concede somewhat, if only to the extent that you can recognize that some of your thoughts are scaring you and that, for now, this is okay.

Is this anxiety familiar to you, or is it a new and unfamiliar expression of your emotional experience? If you have a history of anxious responses, you might feel differently than someone who has never experienced such a high degree of anxiety. Either way, it's disturbing. Consider the following questions:

1. How would you describe your typical emotional response to stress (prior to this current experience)?

   _____
   _____
   _____

2. How is your current experience the same as or different from your previous pattern of emotional responding?

   _____
   _____
   _____

3. Do you think you could learn to tolerate this, even for short periods of time, if you knew, for certain, that nothing bad would happen? Explain why or why not:

_____

_____

_____

Eckhart Tolle teaches us that the conflict between our external circumstances at any given moment and our thoughts and feelings about those circumstances can cause great pain. He asks, "Can you feel how painful it is to internally stand in opposition to what is?" (Tolle, 2003, p. 57)

What *is*, right now, is the presence of thoughts that scare you. The task here is to allow it to be. One helpful technique is the use of affirmations to reduce the internal conflict, such as the following:

- I am having thoughts that scare me.
- I have learned that it's okay that I'm having these thoughts and that nothing bad is happening.
- Good mothers can have scary thoughts.
- Scary thoughts like the ones I am having are extremely common.
- I don't have to like it, but if I acknowledge these thoughts are here, I am taking the first step toward finding relief.
- Thinking something does not make it happen.

Use the space below to repeat these affirmations and/or come up with some of your own that work better for you:

1. _____

2. _____

3. _____

4. _____

5. _____

Identification

Now that you have admitted to yourself that this is happening, the next step is to come face-to-face with some of your thoughts. If you are uncomfortable writing them here, jot them down on a separate sheet of paper that you can destroy afterward, until you feel more prepared to expose how you are feeling or what you are thinking.

Some of the scary thoughts I am having are the following:

1. _____
2. _____
3. _____
4. _____
5. _____

Now, let's break them down further using the categories we have discussed throughout the book (i.e., excessive worry, rumination, obsessive thoughts, intrusive memories, catastrophic misinterpretations of bodily sensations). Do your best to be specific about the details and content of each category that applies to you. Remember that you may have some thoughts in one or two or all categories, or some may be blank. None of that matters. All that matters right now is that you are paying attention to some of the thoughts and trying to view them as cognitive entities without as much emotion attached as you had previously. Remember that the content of your thoughts is not as important as you think. However, identifying the content here will enable you to take a step closer to acceptance, which, ultimately, will bring you peace of mind.

I tend to *worry excessively* about:

1. _____
2. _____
3. _____
4. _____
5. _____

Some of the *ruminations* that go around and around in my head about myself and my internal experiences are:

1. _____
2. _____
3. _____
4. _____
5. _____

My *obsessive thoughts* are mostly about:

1. _____
2. _____
3. _____
4. _____
5. _____

I have these types of *intrusive memories* of my recent labor and delivery or of another trauma:

1. _____
2. _____
3. _____
4. _____
5. _____

I am experiencing these uncomfortable *bodily sensations*, and this is how I am *interpreting* them:

1. _____; _____
2. _____; _____
3. _____; _____
4. _____; _____
5. _____; _____

Disclosure and Barriers

Writing down some of your scary thoughts may have unforeseen therapeutic value. Do not underestimate the power of ridding yourself of some of the discord in your head by displacing it on paper. It will help to release some of the pressure and make room for positive thoughts to balance things out.

Once you can recognize and admit that this is happening, the next step is to identify the obstacles that prevent you from letting others know. Remember that the factors that contribute to the barriers to relief are not absolute givens. They are potential barriers that can be modified, adjusted, or abolished. Once you identify one or more of these barriers that may be impeding your progress, you can begin to make headway through this healing process. Check off any of the following factors that characterize what may be getting in your way of letting others know how you are feeling:

❑ Do you feel unable to distinguish normal postpartum concerns from those that may be problematic? Do you find yourself questioning whether something you are feeling or thinking is "normal" or not?

❑ Do you find that you are your own worst enemy or believe that you are never quite good enough?

❑ Do you find that you often worry about what others will think of you, especially when you feel so vulnerable? Are you worried about being labeled or stereotyped if you talk to someone or reach out for help?

❑ Have you considered the possibility that some of what you are feeling and thinking is a direct result of depressive thinking, which can distort the manner in which you perceive the world around you?

❑ Do you wonder if you are susceptible to the words and viewpoints of others who may or may not have your best interests at heart or who may be misguided by erroneous information?

❑ Do you feel pressure from people around you to feel or behave in certain ways that may inhibit your being totally honest about some of the feelings and thoughts you are having?

❑ Do you find yourself constantly swirling around "what-if" scenarios, bouncing from one troublesome script in your head to another?

Once you have identified some of the factors that may be interfering, make a list of the people you feel *most* comfortable talking to about the thoughts you are having. Next to each name, indicate whether or not you have disclosed to them, and then, why or why not. In other words, try to identify what it is about these people that makes you feel comfortable talking with them about this painful experience.

Name of support person	Yes/no	Why?/why not?

Next, list the people you feel *least* comfortable talking to about the thoughts you are having. Here, identify people with whom you might like to talk, but fear they might not understand or react well, even if you feel you are very close to them and would like to let them in. Again, beside each name, indicate whether you have disclosed to them or not and what, if anything, got in the way.

Name of support person	Yes/no	Why?/why not?

Additional questions to ask yourself:

1. Does everyone have accurate information? In other words, do you think your support people are adequately informed and understand the unique nature of scary thoughts? What might you do to increase the likelihood that they really understand?

   _____

   _____

   _____

2. Do you need to sit down and have a conversation with any of these people and share some of what you have learned so that they have a more complete understanding of what to expect and what all of this means? What are your thoughts about doing this?

   _____

   _____

   _____

The people on the preceding lists may include your partner, your parents, your siblings, your friends, other family members, your doctors, and/or other healthcare providers. Keep in mind that regardless of your relationship, you might be taken aback to discover who is the most compassionate in times like this. It does not always unfold the way you necessarily expect it will.

Be careful not to make assumptions that prohibit you from moving forward, and remember to be clear about what you need. What might that be? Perhaps you want someone to know so that you don't feel so alone. Or, you might want your doctor to know so that you can get a referral to a mental health specialist who can further support you. Or, you might want a friend to understand how scared you are so that she can reassure and comfort you. Or, you might like to fortify your resources in the event that you need more social support while stress is high.

Whatever your reason for disclosing and regardless of how much you are tempted not to do so, remember that there is documented therapeutic value in being able to talk about what you are experiencing and following up with supportive interventions.

You will likely discover that some of the barriers to disclosure are related to your own reluctance, whereas other barriers can be attributed to the people to whom you are considering disclosing or to particular circumstances that may complicate the picture. Understanding which obstacles are attributable to you and which belong to the potential support people should be enlightening. It can help you identify what you need to do about modifying your attitude and approach and what, if anything, you can do to facilitate understanding in those to whom you have reached out.

The following are some frequently asked questions regarding disclosure:

1. *Do I really have to tell someone about my scary thoughts?*

   No, you don't. But as we've discussed, the chances are excellent that you will feel better if you do. The key to lowering your distress through disclosure rests with the person to whom you disclose and the manner in which he or she responds. These factors will largely determine the degree to which you attain relief through telling someone.

2. *What if I tell someone I'm having some scary thoughts, but don't tell them about ALL of my scary thoughts?*

   That's okay. You can hold tight to your "secret" thoughts, but the more you do that, the more likely you are to feel guilty about them. There are no rules as to how to do this. If you think specific details of your thoughts are better left concealed, that's all right. Keep in mind that the content of your thoughts is not as significant as you fear it is.

3. *What if I decide to tell someone and it makes everything worse?*

We sincerely hope that doesn't happen. If it does, then your best recourse is to choose another person from your list and soldier forward in seeking the support you need. Depending on the circumstances that made you believe that disclosing backfired, consider trying to reeducate that person appropriately or waiting until you feel stronger before approaching him or her again.

4. *What if I'm having a scary thought that is not on any of these lists, and I'm certain no one has ever had this despicable thought?*

Someone has. Someone, somewhere, at some time has had a thought similar to the one you're having. The list of thoughts included or referenced in this book is only a partial list. In our clinical practices, women express indescribable relief when they see we are not reactive while they reveal their specific scary thought, no matter how awful it feels to them. Often, they anticipate shock or total disbelief and are calmed when we reassure them it is not the first time we have heard this thought.

Vulnerabilities

The following is a checklist of factors that may increase your risk for scary thoughts. Remember that risk factors do not cause these thoughts, and they do not ensure that you will have them. They are, however, associated with the emergence of scary thoughts, and therefore it may be helpful for you to see what puts you at greatest risk:

Biological vulnerabilities:

❑ I have a personal history of anxiety and/or depression.
❑ I have a family history of anxiety and/or depression.
❑ I have always been inclined to be emotional around my period or have a history of moderate to severe PMS.

❑ I have a history of responding well to medications for anxiety and/or depression.

❑ I have blood relatives who have responded well to medications for anxiety and/or depression.

❑ I recently gave birth, which means my hormone levels have not returned to normal.

❑ I am breastfeeding.

Psychological vulnerabilities:

❑ I have trouble coping with ambiguous or uncertain situations.

❑ I believe that worrying will help me or protect me or my baby from harm.

❑ I lack confidence in my ability to solve problems.

❑ I avoid thinking about images of potential catastrophes.

❑ I have a tendency to ruminate or beat myself up when things aren't going well.

❑ I believe that thinking about bad or scary thoughts increases the likelihood that they will occur.

❑ I believe that thinking about bad or scary thoughts is equivalent to acting on them.

❑ I believe that the cost of having bad or scary thoughts is extraordinary.

❑ I believe that I am responsible for preventing bad or scary thoughts from happening.

❑ I believe that I must control bad or scary thoughts that come into my mind.

❑ I am a perfectionist.

❑ I have had trouble coping with adversity in the past.

❑ I lack confidence in my ability to cope with adversity.

❑ I have a tendency to become anxious when I experience physical or emotional symptoms of anxiety.

❑ In the past, I have catastrophized about the implications of bodily sensations that I experienced.

It doesn't matter how many of these items you have checked off. Recognize that checking any of these will increase your risk for scary thoughts. But, again, because almost *all* mothers have scary thoughts, it shouldn't surprise you if you checked many or all of the risk factors. If you checked off statements in the first group, you have some vulnerabilities that make you a good candidate for biological support, and medications may help you feel better. If you checked more in the second group, you are likely to respond well to psychotherapy.

Understanding your particular areas of vulnerability will facilitate a clearer picture of how you can best help yourself and the most appropriate ways to intervene. Women rarely fit neatly into one category, so most women will check some items from both groups. Because every woman is unique, we again emphasize that if you do not like the way you are feeling, it is best to seek professional support. Healthcare professionals in the field are most equipped to help you navigate through this often confusing and emotional time.

Self-Help and Nonprofessional Interventions

The following are the self-help strategies that we described in Chapter 7 as being effective tools for coping with scary thoughts. The questions and exercises will help you determine the strategies that would be most beneficial to you.

Avoiding Pitfalls

❑ Are you pretending or acting as if you are not having scary thoughts?
❑ Are you trying to force your scary thoughts from your mind only to have them return full strength?
❑ Do you find yourself responding to your scary thoughts with irrational fear?

Keeping Your Brain Busy

List some of the feel-good activities in which you generally engage that help distract you from your thoughts, even if only for a short while (e.g., reading, watching TV, walking, calling a friend, journaling, crossword puzzles, listening to music):

_____

_____

_____

_____

_____

_____

1. What is your go-to, single most reliable distraction technique that has worked in the past and continues to be effective when you are most anxious?

   _____

2. Is this technique working for you now? If not, why do you think it is not?

   _____

3. What activities do you think you could add that might help at this point (see examples in Chapter 7). Remember that the more you find to keep your brain busy, the less energy you will have to worry, ruminate, and obsess.

   _____
   _____
   _____
   _____
   _____
   _____

Just Breathe

Can you set aside 30 minutes a day for yourself? What about 20 minutes? Or 5 minutes? Even if you cannot carve out time that is specifically designed for relaxation, breathing, or mindfulness exercises, it will nonetheless be helpful to concentrate on controlling and relaxing your breathing throughout the day, such as when you are sitting at the computer, talking on the phone, driving, resting, watching TV, or working.

The mistake that many postpartum women make is that they consider this to be a luxury. It is not. Taking care of yourself is an essential priority. Make time for it. See if you can set 5–10 minutes each day for 2 weeks to sit, clear your head, and breathe, relax, and/or practice mindfulness. If this exercise makes you feel more anxious, do not do it until you feel it can be helpful. When you can, check off each day that you treat yourself to this as you build toward greater self-control and peacefulness. Documenting this exercise makes you accountable, which generally leads to greater compliance.

	Breathing	**Relaxation**	**Mindfulness**
Monday	_____	_____	_____
Tuesday	_____	_____	_____
Wednesday	_____	_____	_____
Thursday	_____	_____	_____
Friday	_____	_____	_____
Saturday	_____	_____	_____
Sunday	_____	_____	_____

S.E.L.F Care (Sleep, Exercise, Laughter, Food)

List one thing after each S.E.L.F. item that you can do differently to augment your self-care regime:

❑ Are you getting adequate sleep? If not, what do you think is getting in the way? What steps are you taking to remedy this?

_____

_____

❑ Are you getting adequate exercise? If not, are you getting out of the house and walking a block or two so that you can move your muscles and begin to reap the benefits?

_____

_____

❑ Are you able to access any moments of pure fun or laughter? If not, can you go out of your way to find something that can tickle your funny bone for the sake of your mental and spiritual well-being?

_____

_____

❑ Are you avoiding caffeine, alcohol, and excessive sugar? Are you eating well-balanced meals and snacks? If not, can you take steps to introduce fruits, vegetables, nuts, protein, and whole grains into your diet so that you can see if it helps you feel better and think more clearly?

_____

_____

Nonprofessional Interventions

Have you tried any of these nonprofessional interventions that have been shown to be helpful?

❏ Self-help books or audio/video tape materials
❏ Journaling
❏ Support groups
❏ Online support
❏ Omega-3 fish oil supplements
❏ Light therapy

Cognitive Strategies

Think back to Chapter 8, when we proposed that one of the most direct ways to modify scary thoughts is to evaluate their accuracy and helpfulness systematically. We encouraged you to construct balanced responses to your scary thoughts when you found them to be associated with emotional distress. Use this opportunity to indicate which cognitive strategies worked best for you:

❏ Scary Thought Log
❏ Experiment
❏ Coping card
❏ Discussion with a "coach"

If the Scary Thought Log was helpful for you, record the questions that were most effective in helping you to evaluate your scary thoughts:
1. _____
2. _____
3. _____

If the Scary Thought Log was helpful for you, record the balanced responses you constructed that were most compelling and effective in reducing your emotional distress:
1. _____
2. _____
3. _____

If you tried an experiment, what did you learn from it?

1. _____
2. _____
3. _____

If you made one or more coping cards, where will you keep it/them?

_____

If you decided that it would be best to evaluate scary thoughts with another person, who will serve as your "coach"?

_____

Did you experience any problems in using the cognitive strategies? If so, what were they?

1. _____
2. _____
3. _____

How can you overcome those problems?

_____

_____

If you use a combination of the self-help strategies described in Chapter 7 and the cognitive strategies described in Chapter 8, what is the most effective way to implement them systematically when you identify a scary thought?

_____

_____

Professional Treatment Options

Most women have a long list of concerns regarding medication and/or psychotherapy during the postpartum period. Consider these questions as you navigate this decision-making process:

1. How much do you think stigma and the associated shame and self-blame are still getting in the way of your getting help for the way you are feeling?

   _____

   _____

2. If you have ever had any treatment for anxiety or depression, including medication and/or psychotherapy of any kind, list them here:

   _____

   _____

   _____

3. If so, were they helpful? Which were most and least helpful? Why or why not?

   _____

   _____

   _____

4. What is your view about taking medication for anxiety and/or depression right now if you need it?

   _____

   _____

5. Under what specific conditions would you consider taking medication if a trusted healthcare provider indicated that it might be helpful?

   _____

   _____

6. If you are breastfeeding, what steps do you need to take to proceed with adequate information and support?

   _____

   _____

7. Has anyone in your family been helped by medication for anxiety or depression?

   _____

   _____

8. What is your view about going to psychotherapy for anxiety and/or depression?

_____

_____

_____

9. If you have had psychotherapy in the past, was it helpful? In what ways was it most helpful or why do you think it was not?

_____

_____

_____

10. Do you believe your partner will be supportive of any decision you make regarding professional treatment options? Why or why not?

_____

_____

11. Using the following scale, rate your distress regarding the thoughts you are having:

```
|____|____|____|____|____|____|____|____|____|____|
 0    1    2    3    4    5    6    7    8    9   10
Least distress                            Worst distress I
                                          have ever felt
```

What number would you rate your emotional distress right now?

_____

How bad does your distress need to feel before you decide to seek treatment? _____

12. What are your most pressing concerns about medication or psychotherapy?

_____

_____

13. Who are your best (objective, reliable, trustworthy, supportive) contacts to help you make a decision regarding treatment options?

_____

_____

_____

14. What do you see as your biggest barrier to getting the treatment you might need right now? What do you think you might need to do about that?

_____

_____

Acceptance

As we approach the end of this book, it will be helpful for you to continue to pay close attention to your innermost thoughts and emotions. Only you know what you are really feeling, what you are really most afraid of, and what may be getting in your way. It's hard to be brutally honest when you feel broken inside. Sometimes the fear of putting words out there, either on paper or in dialogue, can be greater than the original fear itself. Try to be gentle with yourself as you take charge of how you are feeling and what you need. You have done a great deal of work here. You have dared to confront a part of yourself that was in position to challenge the essence of who you are. You should feel proud of the efforts you have made to acknowledge and accept the presence of such contrary emotions and thoughts. In the final chapter, we will see how motherhood will continue to test you and how you can best stay focused, how you can allow your anxiety just to be, and how to continue to feel healthy.

Take-Home Point for Mothers. The workbook format of this chapter will help you monitor how you are feeling and determine the steps that need to be taken to achieve a state of acceptance so that you can feel better. You can choose to share the contents of this chapter with your partner, your therapist, or your friend. Or, you can use it as a private diary for your own edification.

Clinician Note. The chapter will serve as a useful tool to enable you to walk through some of the personal resources and biases that may either augment or impede your client's acceptance and recovery process.

12

Living With Uncertainty

Motherhood has been the subject of scholarly and creative writing for centuries. There is much written on the demands, the exhilaration, the drama, and the formidable task of adjusting to the onslaught of challenges. Along with the joys that accompany the transition to this major event in a woman's life, motherhood may also be a stressful experience that generates intense anxiety and pervasive feelings of incompetence and loneliness.

Still, only recently have mothers, researchers, and clinicians come forward to address the alarming nature of maternal musings. We have discussed that unsettling and unwanted thoughts can emerge on a continuum of tolerance: Some are experienced as a nuisance, whereas others torment a mother's mind until she believes she is most certainly going mad. When this happens, the associated distress and scary thoughts permeate the very air she breathes.

As we conclude this book, let us consider two final points that pulse at the heart of this issue. Understanding anxiety within the context of motherhood can evoke both controversy and earnest sentiment. Many renowned writers have made the case for more stringent societal acceptance of the rampant anxiety and demands of motherhood. Judith Warner even went so far as to label it a *perfect madness* (2005). As she states in her book with this title:

> [This book] is an explanation of a feeling. That caught-by-the-throat feeling that so many mothers have today that they are *always* doing something wrong. And it's about this conviction I have that this feeling—this widespread, choking cocktail of guilt and anxiety and resentment and regret—is poisoning motherhood for American women today. (Warner, 2005, p. 4)

Warner holds numerous factions accountable for this current genera-
tion of mothers under pressure—from media-soaked promises of absolute
excellence to feministic declarations of grand achievements. The claim
that mothers are sentenced to this state of chronic discontent paints a
bleak picture, to be sure. Furthermore, if mothers are already feeling con-
demned to standards of perfection by society, by their friends, by family,
and by themselves, how can they ever be expected to free themselves from
the "existential anxiety" that ubiquitously controls their every move? Not
a comforting thought.

Adding to this frenzy is a second consideration: the concept of trait
anxiety. This concept refers to the intrinsic tendency to react with anxiety
across a number of situations and different times throughout a person's life.
Jerome Kagan, a Harvard professor of psychology, spent years researching
the way in which a baby's innate temperament impacts a person's development over time (Kagan & Snidman, 2009). He discovered that babies
who are highly reactive tend to grow up anxious and concluded that some
people are predisposed to this highly reactive state and are, quite simply,
born anxious. A recent *New York Times* review of Kagan's somewhat con-
troversial work highlighted the point that "some people, no matter how
robust their stock portfolios or how healthy their children, are always
mentally preparing for doom. They are just born worriers, their brains
forever anticipating the dropping of some dreaded other shoe." (Henig,
2009, para. 8)

When we consider the implications of trait anxiety in postpartum women,
we find women who are consistently putting forth their best efforts and, at
the same time, think they are never doing quite enough. Some women are
born anxious. Some babies have highly reactive temperaments.

Ultimately, a mother can only do her best.

Of course, some experts might argue that this notion of trait anxiety is
in direct conflict with the assertion of developmental psychologists that
each of us is born with a blank slate and environmental influences reign
supreme. For instance, the philosophy of attachment parenting promotes
the belief that emotional sensitivity and physical closeness are the underlying principle behind developmental health: *Stay in close contact to your
baby, breastfeed with skin-to-skin contact, and wear the baby with you so
that he can hear your heartbeat.* Although no one disputes the power of the
mother–child bond and its impact on future development, Kagan claims
that a child's temperament, which is inherited and potentially linked to

certain sets of emotions and behaviors, can be only slightly influenced by the parents (Kagan & Snidman 2009). This is the precise point that makes his theory divisive.

The debate of nature versus nurture is not new. The relevance here is that, depending on one's frame of reference, mothers could conceivably be taking on way too much responsibility for things that may be largely out of their control. Consider the mother who has made a secure attachment with her baby, who possesses a high-reactive temperament. This child may be challenging and difficult to soothe, prompting the mother to assume unjust blame. Interestingly, the message here is twofold: Mothers should not undeservedly blame themselves for the disposition of their baby and they should not blame themselves for their own heightened degree of anxiety, which may or may not be an intrinsic tendency.

If we combine the *perfect madness* (Warner, 2005) of the enduring societal pressure cooker with the notion of inherited predispositions of some women to be more anxious than others, we find a volatile condition looming in the shadows. We, as a society and as individuals, need to recalibrate expectations in order to alleviate the continuous and unnecessary self-blame, guilt, and liability that mothers assume for things beyond their control.

Motherhood, as we have seen, is a period in life that is fraught with unpredictability and crushing uncertainties. It seems that no matter how hard they try or how quickly they move, mothers cannot outrun their cascading worries and scary thoughts. Yet, armed with information and support, mothers can indeed discover the protection they seek. We are aware that, at first glance, these views create a rather gloomy portrayal of so-called maternal bliss. Still, it is possible—and the primary intent of this book—to distract you from the temptation to surrender to the forces that hold you back from experiencing joy and to empower you with the tools to do so.

ADAPTIVE AWARENESS

Recognizing and understanding your own anxiety might mean the difference between unnecessary suffering and healthy coping. Consider the very real possibility that if you are not able or refuse to acknowledge that you even have anxiety, you may be destined to feel overwhelmed and out-matched by the dangers of an unpredictable world. If, on the other hand, you are able to identify and label your anxiety, rather than attribute the heightened fear to the magnitude of the situation itself, you will be better prepared to take action that could potentially minimize your unsettling feelings. This is generally true, but it is categorically true with regard to scary thoughts. Conversely, if you deny your anxiety, you are more likely to exaggerate the perceived threat and feel utterly powerless.

Recall Elizabeth from Chapter 1, who struggled with obsessive thoughts and images. She was familiar with the concept of scary thoughts but felt no less frustrated by her own scary thoughts after the birth of her second child. She felt prepared for her second baby and was surprised when she was let down by her husband this time around. Though he tried, repeatedly, to say all the right things and shower her with reassurance, Elizabeth found herself continuously dragged by the riptide. Once more she found herself treading water alone in what she called her "black lonely place." She thought she knew what she was up against, yet she couldn't fight the surge of the tide.

Telling someone to be aware of her own anxiety is like telling someone in the middle of a panic attack to relax. It doesn't feel good to hear, and it certainly doesn't seem like it can help. Typically, if a therapist were to point out to an anxious client that she should become aware of her anxiety, the therapist might be met with: *Are you kidding me?! That's ALL I'm aware of. How 'bout helping me become LESS aware of my anxiety?!* Hyperawareness comes with the territory of anxiety, as we've seen throughout this book

The awareness we now refer to as part of the healing process is slightly different. It occurs as a learned coping response to anxiety and is a state of acute consciousness in which you recognize the existence of the anxiety while simultaneously detaching from it, as if you were on the outside looking in. Ideally, the awareness will precede the anxiety. That is, if you are aware that you tend to be anxious, you are more likely to respond thoughtfully, rather than being frightened by your reactions and feelings. This adaptive awareness allows you to view the anxiety as an integral part of yourself while, at the same time, being less likely to let it overwhelm you. For some, learning to identify the negative inner monologue and to reframe it can successfully lead the way to the development of healthy coping strategies.

Elizabeth worked hard to reverse old patterns and create a new script on which she could rely each time she felt bombarded by a thought that scared her.

- This is a scary thought.
- This is not real.
- My mind is playing a trick on me.
- I need to stop and do something else.

Elizabeth became more aware of her tendency to surrender to her obsessive thoughts and images, and she developed skills that allowed her to intervene on her own behalf. Understanding that her scary thoughts were irrational gave her the distance she needed to rally against them. She repeated this soliloquy over and over each time she was confronted with an unwanted thought or image. Increased awareness allowed Elizabeth the option to respond differently, and every time she did so, it allowed the new pattern to be engraved a bit more securely in her mind.

Your increased awareness will bring you closer to a sense of your true self. This may sound like a cliché or overly simplistic, but if anxiety and the presence of scary thoughts are part of your life right now, embracing this fact is far more constructive than hating it and wishing it away. Being aware of your vulnerabilities provides valuable information and prepares you to cope with the inevitable ebbs and flows of motherhood.

LIVING WITH THE UNPREDICTABILITY OF MOTHERHOOD

There is great value in learning to live with some of the anxiety that comes with motherhood. Once you identify the mechanism that rests behind scary thoughts, you begin to see it everywhere. Anxiety is sprinkled throughout every typical day. From an inconsolable baby to insufficient sleep to a genetic predisposition, anxiety during motherhood is much more the norm than the exception. In fact, there is nothing terribly remarkable about mothers and anxiety other than to say that it is so very routine and rather unexceptional. That is, of course, except when anxiety is extreme, severe, or debilitating; such can be the case with the anxiety that is linked to scary thoughts. Mothers need to feel better prepared for this common but frightening experience.

We know that scary thoughts are universal, and we understand that anxiety will thrive, whether or not it is welcomed. Therefore, it follows that the best course of action is to accept these realities and simultaneously cultivate a greater sense of resiliency as backup. *Resiliency* refers to the capacity to bounce back from adversity or to endure hardship of some kind, and it takes time to develop and fortify. Still, each step you make in this direction enables you to protect yourself better against the uncertainties that lie ahead:

- **Accept the current state.** In Chapter 7, we briefly explored the concept of accepting the current state of your distress. Resisting what is occurring is a sure-fire way to increase your anxiety, frustration, fear, and a host of other undesirable emotional responses. As we've seen, accepting the current state is difficult to do if you are accustomed to thinking negatively. Still, this fundamental first step lays the groundwork for acceptance and inner strength.
- **Take care of yourself and your relationships.** Everyone wrestles with her own demons from time to time. Those times when you feel the very least desire to reach out are often the times when it is most important for you to do so. The ability to connect with yourself, your partner, and others is a vital aspect of healing. Resiliency comes from connection, not isolation.
- **Recognize your own strengths.** Perhaps it's hard to think about the gifts you bring to others and what it is about you that others admire or need, but reclaiming your self-esteem is exactly what you need to do. Have you lost sight of what distinguishes you from others? Are you taking yourself for granted because you are so tired of being anxious and scared of your own thoughts? Are you aware that it's possible to be anxious and competent at the same time? Postpartum women, who are working hard to be perfect, forget that they can be symptomatic and strong simultaneously. Many mistakenly presume that if they have symptoms, they are weak. Again, accept the current state of distress and continue to be strong and move forward through this.
- **Set limits.** This a time when it is crucial to learn how to say no. Equally relevant is when and to what you say yes. Are you making

yourself too available? Are you worried about what others might think? Establishing appropriate boundaries will help you reserve strength and minimize burnout. Anxiety eats up enormous amounts of energy; setting limits can help you refuel.

- **Find your sense of humor.** If you've lost your sense of humor, try to find it. If you're not sure whether you ever had one or not, surround yourself with people who make you laugh or feel good. Everyone knows that good, hearty laughter is contagious. Force yourself to get out of your head and find a funny place to rest for a while. It distracts your brain from its scary thoughts while, at the same time, helping you breathe more deeply. Humor helps you break through the boundaries imposed upon you by your scary thoughts, if only for a moment, and frees you from the perceived seriousness of the situation. Coping becomes more bearable when things feel lighter.

- **Forgive yourself and others.** Be gentle with yourself and your tender spots; you have seen that you are vulnerable in ways that may predispose you to distress. Kindness, tolerance, and forgiveness are the cornerstone of acceptance and emotional well-being. We have discussed that opposition to the current state of anxiety does little more than regenerate anxiety. Begin to believe that you can endure this high state of anxiety without judgment, without fear of recrimination, without blame. Believe that you are struggling with something that has a name and a clinical course that responds to treatment. You are not doomed to be at the mercy of your unwanted thoughts. You have learned a great deal and can continue to stretch beyond your instinct to run and hide. Recognize your achievements along the way and reward yourself for facing and speaking the truth.

- **Find meaning.** How you respond to life's challenges largely depends on your resiliency. Submitting to the pain and powerlessness of unwanted thoughts will leave you feeling weak and disheartened. The wisdom that comes from breaking the cycle of scary thoughts involves the capacity to reinterpret this negative experience. How can you find meaning from such agony? That is the pearl that you must discover on your own because it is uniquely your experience. As futile as it may feel, finding the meaning in any crisis builds resilience by elevating your spirit. You can try to resist the temptation to view your experience as only negative. Inherent in each of us is the desire to make sense out of our lives, particularly those moments that make no sense at all. Finding meaning to scary thoughts may sound preposterous. But the key to resilience and adaptation is the ability to do just that—the ability to reconstruct the negative framework into something that makes more sense. (*This anxiety felt unbearable at times, but it enabled me to learn more about myself and how I cope, so I can do it differently in the future.*) In this way, you attribute a purpose to these events and the life lesson propels you further forward.

MASTERY

Virtually every mother, at one point or another, has battled scary thoughts, images, or impulses. Trapped by their increasing emotional distress, mothers often have trouble understanding the nature of these unwanted thoughts and urges. They may be embroiled in cultural beliefs that do not tolerate a mother's failure to exude unconditional love, or they may struggle mightily and torture themselves with relentless self-blame. They mistakenly try to measure their maternal success by the absence of distress. They may feel pressure amid the array of supportive voices clamoring around them or from their own self-persecuting whispers. For all mothers, the hard truth is that anxiety is part of the package. Accepting the awesome reality that motherhood is indeed laden with angst is the first step toward understanding and managing the anxiety that emerges.

As you continue to review your experience, both in your life and in this book, our hope is that you have acquired new skills and insight into your experience with scary thoughts and the emotional distress that they cause. We trust that this leaves you feeling better equipped to evaluate these thoughts and to seek support or professional guidance so that you can suffer less and experience greater joy. In the end, it's important that you acknowledge and accept that scary thoughts are manifestations of distress and not your fault. Nor are they an indication that something bad is going to happen. As you proceed through this process of living with your anxiety and taking care of it at the same time, you will minimize your sense of helplessness and maximize your sense of empowerment.

It is always difficult to face and endure painful emotions. It is particularly difficult when these emotions accompany the life-altering and spectacular changes that take place during motherhood. But as you continue to improve your ability to manage your anxiety, you will achieve a new sense of mastery over what once felt insurmountable. You will see that as you accept your distressing emotions, positive emotions begin to surface. You will soon discover bits of joyfulness reentering your life, often when you least expect it.

Afterword

For the last 20 years, I have planned, promised myself, and intended to write a book about perinatal mood disorders. Karen Kleiman does not plan, promise, or intend. Karen Kleiman writes books. She is, perhaps, the most prolific and most recognized writer on the subject. Karen and I have "known" each other for about 15 years; yet, we actually met just a few years ago. The bond was instantaneous. We've traveled many of the same paths. We can say, unabashedly, that we are pioneers within this "movement" of awareness, consciousness raising, training, and educating the public on what was once an unrecognized, overlooked, and misdiagnosed illness. We figured out how to treat depressed and frightened moms at all levels of distress. We were there when the rumblings began. Barely perceptible. No Internet. No e-mail. Slowly, the connections and the weaving began. The rumblings grew louder and became stronger. Organizations began to emerge. We found Depression After Delivery (DAD) and Postpartum Support International (PSI). Newsletters and articles began to appear. We received them via snail mail.

Like most of us involved in the postpartum "movement," I am a survivor. It was 1980. I was truly enjoying my pregnancy. I absolutely loved the attention and the movement in my belly. Strangers let you ahead of them in lines. They help with heavy packages. They gave themselves permission to touch your belly. While some women objected, I never minded that boundary being crossed. Somewhere around the eighth month of my pregnancy, it reality hit: This baby has to come out of me. It truly was a different time. Painkillers were shunned because they would be harmful to the baby. The only way to go was "natural." Some 22 years later, I read Naomi Wolf's book, *Misconceptions,* and came across this African proverb:

> Being pregnant and giving birth are like crossing a narrow bridge. People can accompany you to the bridge. They can greet you on the other side. But you walk that bridge alone.

This proverb—this metaphor—has stayed with me all these years. We all encounter bridges of various types, lengths, and strengths as we travel through our lives: adolescence, leaving home for the first time, and marriage, to name a few.

I'd like to share with you three bridges I have crossed and continue to cross. These three bridges are structurally quite similar. I imagine them to be primitive suspension bridges made of wood planks and rope. A pair of supports at either end (trees, stakes, or poles) secure the bridge. Wood poles are intermittently bored through the wood planks along the bridge to secure the length of rope to which the traveler holds as he or she makes his or her way to the other side. Beneath the bridge lie sharp rocks and turbulent waters.

Back to my own personal experiences: Bridge number one, pregnancy, was rather fun. The bridge was sturdy. I walked across with great confidence. But as I got closer to the other side, thoughts of labor and delivery began to permeate my brain. I froze. I had nightmares of being sliced open. I had nightmares of a "natural" delivery. I had nightmares of dying on the table. There was no escape and the bridge began to wobble.

"The hell with Lamaze classes. This is going to hurt. A lot." Of course I had the option of the much frowned upon painkillers, but that would make me a childbirth failure and a bad mother before even leaving the delivery room. Surely medication would harm my baby in some way. Could I ever forgive myself? What would others think? But I saw all those women on the other side of the bridge, supporting and encouraging me—since the beginning of time.

"If they could do it, I can do it." So, with the help of a shot of Demerol (took *years* to forgive myself for that one) and nearly 15 hours of labor (I think the number of hours get longer every year), I crossed that bridge with my son in my arms. I was greeted with excitement and joy. I was carried on their shoulders like the MVP after a football game. Then, I was back on the ground and they slowly drifted away. The fanfare was over. I quickly learned that labor doesn't end in the delivery room.

My son was a preemie, born 1 month prior to his due date. His skin seemed nearly translucent and hung from his body like that on a raw chicken. Colic began within a few days—no respecter of day or night. It didn't take long for it to reset my inner clock and for the insomnia to set in. I'm anxious. I'm depressed. I'm immobilized. I'm exhausted. I can't seem to do anything right. My baby hates me.

There is no support whatsoever. My own undoing, I'm a master of disguise. Besides, I had a reputation of being strong and competent. I had an image to maintain. I told no one. You know the drill: shame, embarrassment, guilt, and fear. Obviously, my (ex) husband was aware of the insomnia and my uncontrollable crying. Each day he'd come home from work and see me in the same shapeless housedress. I engaged in little to no self-care and was totally isolated. My husband's initial show of concern soon turned to annoyance. I'll never forget the day he came home from work and pulled the dress off my shoulders and threw it in the garbage. He just didn't get it. Neither did I. He became more and more distant and unavailable. Today, we recognize that men can have postpartum depression, too.

I approach bridge number two. I am surrounded by "seasoned" moms who have frequently offered me well meaning but unsolicited advice. They contradict one another. They confuse me and add to my mounting sense of inadequacy. But now, everything is OK. I can see the sign as I stand before the bridge: "Motherhood Straight Ahead." It is framed with cherubs and fluffy white clouds. It's going to be a long walk, but when I squint, I can see all the beautiful, blissful mothers nursing, nurturing, and nuzzling their newborn babies on the other side. The babies are content and cooing sweetly. I want that.

I take my first tentative step. Baby in one arm, hand of the other grasping the rope. Clearly, this is going to be a challenge. This bridge is not the same as the first. The slats are faded and worn. The links connecting the slats are rusted. The ropes are frayed. This bridge wobbles and sways as the wind whips up. The water below is turbulent. In addition to my baby, I am carrying all the symptoms I had before I embarked upon this new journey.

However, there is now a new dimension: *What if my baby falls from my arm? What if he is swept away by the waters below? What if he is crushed by the rocks? What if we both topple over?* I can see it all in my mind's eye. Other thoughts—intrusive thoughts, each one more horrific than the last—leave me shaken and gasping for air. I would *never* harm my child. The depression deepens and the anxiety turns to terror; I am thoroughly exhausted. I am holding on to that rope for dear life. I take that final step off that bridge and am now surrounded by the serene and peaceful images I saw when I squinted at the beginning of this journey.

I made it! But not really. I am not like them. I'm different. There is something wrong with me. I am as unsteady and as unstable as the bridge I just crossed. I need to sit and rest. I find a shady tree. Propped up, baby on my arm, I close my eyes. At last, some respite. I drift off. But not for long.

Here come those images again. They are vivid, tragic, and revolting. I am startled into awareness; I sit up abruptly and, once again, I am gasping for air.

The jig is up, the mask is off, and I am desperate for help. I find an older, kindly female psychiatrist and tell her about my depression, anxiety, and, worst of all, insomnia. No mention of intrusive thoughts and how they exacerbated my sleep disturbance. I am diagnosed with "major depression," given a prescription for an antidepressant, and sent on my way. The medicine did work. Sleep did come and, with time, the thoughts began to drift away.

Some 4 years later, by a sheer luck, I come across an article in a magazine about "postpartum depression" (PPD). I call the author (founder of Depression After Delivery) and find enormous relief. I was never really alone. I "suffered in silence" like hundreds of thousands of women in the United States every year. They, too, did not come forward due to shame and embarrassment. (Note: By now, my son is 4 and my daughter is a newborn—by the grace of God, the PPD following her birth was mild in comparison.)

The networking began. *The New Mother Syndrome*, by Carol Dix, was published in 1988, 8 years after my trauma. The book was informative and validating. As a social worker in the helping profession, I knew I had to enlighten others. My "lectures" began in the living rooms of childbirth instructors, then hospitals, and then large organizations. By now, I have established The Center for Postpartum Adjustment, and the moms begin to trickle in for counseling and psychotherapy. I am flying by the seat of my pants because there is no script or manual for treating this population. I am my own frame of reference. The common threads begin to emerge: the symptoms, the myths, the unrealistic expectations. We discuss grief and loss associated with becoming a parent. Their "normal negative feelings" are validated. I learn to ask the hard questions: "Do you think you will harm yourself or your baby?" "Are you having scary thoughts?" They know they are safe and accepted.

It's been 30 years. I am 56 years old. I have treated thousands of women and have been blessed with a wonderful reputation in a very large community. I've got my treatment techniques down pat: cognitive therapy, interpersonal therapy, and Ilyene Barsky therapy (aka "gut feeling"). Thanks to Karen Kleiman's new book, *Therapy and the Postpartum Woman*, clinicians now have a "how to" manual. I am also the longest standing member of Postpartum Support International, a worldwide organization working toward the eradication of ignorance surrounding perinatal mood disorders. I have been their Florida coordinator and volunteered in numerous capacities for many years. I have lived to see this illness in scholarly journals and books, in TV plots, and as the subject of public service announcements. I have lived to see women routinely screened by their medical providers and the passage of The Mothers Act. I am enormously proud of the role I have played. I will be leaving my footprint.

I just learned 6 months ago that I am standing in front of my final bridge. Many other bridges have come and gone, but it is this third bridge I'd like to share with you. It is strong and sturdy.

My husband, Mark, has seen to it that this bridge is safe. He has replaced the old slats with new ones. No more rusty links. The rope is taut and secure. I am sad, but not afraid. I look behind me and see my greatest legacy of all: my children. I have lived to watch them cross their own bridges with style and grace and their own personal flair. Gavin, now 30, and Monica, now 26, allow me to go on this final journey with peace. They are college grads, working on their careers, and will be self-sufficient. They are genuinely good, warm, caring people. The best part of my life? Being their mother. In fact, despite turbulent beginnings, I have been an *awesome* mother!

I do believe that my own mother and father will be there to greet me on the other side. I know they have been watching over me and are proud of me, too. I hope my beloved childhood dog is with them. I believe we will all appear to each other as we were when we were last together, but before we became ill. I suspect I will be tired by the time I reach them and will want to rest. I remember, as a child, falling asleep in one room and waking up in another. They carried me. I am still their child and they will carry me again.

I do not know how long it will take me to cross this bridge. Who does? But I will be OK. Remember what I said at the beginning of this afterword? Despite the oxymoron, I am a survivor.

Kol haolam kulo gesher tsar meod v'haikkar lo lefached klol (Hebrew) Translation: The entire world is a narrow bridge. The main thing is not to fear.

Ilyene Barsky, MSW
The Center for Postpartum Adjustment

References

Abramowitz, J. S., Khandker, M., Nelson, C. A., Deacon, B. J., & Rygwall, R. (2006). The role of cognitive factors in obsessive-compulsive symptoms: A prospective study. *Behaviour Research and Therapy, 44,* 1361–1374.

Abramowitz, J. S., Nelson, C. A., Rygwall, R., & Khandker, M. (2007). The cognitive mediation of obsessive-compulsive symptoms: A longitudinal study. *Journal of Anxiety Disorders, 21,* 91–104.

Abramowitz, J. S., Schwartz, S. A., & Moore K. M. (2003). Obsessional thoughts in postpartum females and their partners: Content, severity, and relationship with depression. *Journal of Clinical Psychology in Medical Settings, 10,* 157–164.

Abramowitz, J. S., Schwartz, S. A., Moore, K. M., & Luenzmann, K. R. (2003). Obsessive-compulsive symptoms in pregnancy and the puerperium: A review of the literature. *Journal of Anxiety Disorders, 17,* 461–478.

Aldao, A., Nolen-Hoeksema, S., & Schweizer, S. (2010). Emotion-regulation strategies across psychopathology: A meta-analytic review. *Clinical Psychology Review, 30,* 217–237.

Allen, S. (1998). A qualitative analysis of the process, mediating variables, and impact of traumatic childbirth. *Journal of Reproductive and Infant Psychology, 16,* 107–131.

Altemus, M. (2001). Obsessive-compulsive disorder during pregnancy and postpartum. In K. Yonkers & B. Little (Eds.), *Management of psychiatric disorders in pregnancy* (pp. 149–163). New York, NY: Oxford University Press.

Amankwaa, L. (2003). Postpartum depression among African-American women. *Issues in Mental Health Nursing, 24,* 297–316.

American Congress of Obstetricians and Gynecologists, (2009). Postpartum depression is top priority for new ACOG president. Retrieved January 10, 2010, from www.acog.org/from_home/publications/press_releases/nr05-06-09-1.cfm

American Psychiatric Association. (2000). *Diagnostic and statistical manual of mental disorders* (4th ed.). Text revision. Washington, DC: Author.

Amstadter, A. B., Nugent, N. R., & Koenen, K. C. (2009). Genetics of PTSD: Fear conditioning as a model for future research. *Psychiatric Annals, 39,* 358–367.

Areias, M. E., Kumar, R., Barros, H., & Figueiredo, E. (1996). Correlates of postnatal depression in mothers and fathers. *British Journal of Psychiatry, 169,* 36–41.

Armstrong, K., & Edwards, H. (2003). The effects of exercise and social support on mothers reporting depressive symptoms: A pilot randomized controlled trial. *International Journal of Mental Health Nursing, 12,* 130–138.

Austin, D. W., & Richards, J. C. (2001). The catastrophic misinterpretation model of panic disorder. *Behaviour Research and Therapy, 39,* 1277–1291.

Austin, M-P, Tully L., & Parker, G. (2007). Examining the relationship between antenatal anxiety and postnatal depression. *Journal of Affective Disorders, 101,* 169–174.

Baer, L. (2001). *The imp of the mind.* London, England: Penguin Books.

Bailham, D., & Joseph, S. (2003) Post-traumatic stress following childbirth: A review of the emerging literature and directions for research and practice. *Psychology, Health and Medicine, 8,* 159–167.

Barr, J., & Beck, C. (2008). Infanticide secrets: Qualitative study on postpartum depression. *Canadian Family Physician, 54,* 1716–1717.

Beck, A. T., Rush, A. J., Shaw, B. F., & Emery, G. (1979). *Cognitive therapy of depression.* New York, NY: Guilford.

Beck, C. T., & Driscoll, J. W. (2006). *Postpartum mood and anxiety disorders: A clinician's guide.* Boston, MA: Jones and Bartlett.

Beck, C. T., & Gable, R. (2000). Postpartum depression screening scale: Development and psychometric testing. *Nursing Research, 49,* 272–282.

Beck, J. S. (1995). *Cognitive therapy: Basics and beyond.* New York, NY: Guilford.

Berk, L. S., Tan, S. A., Fry, W. F., Jr., Napier, B. J., Lee, J. W., Hubbard, R. W., & Lewis, J. E. (1989). Neuroendocrine and stress hormone changes during mirthful laughter. *American Journal of the Medical Sciences, 298,* 390–396.

Bleiberg, K. L., & Markowitz, J. C. (2005). A pilot study of interpersonal psychotherapy for posttraumatic stress disorder. *American Journal of Psychiatry, 162,* 181–183.

Borkovec, T. D., & Inz, J. (1990).The nature of worry in generalized anxiety disorder: A predominance of thought activity. *Behaviour Research and Therapy, 28,* 153–158.

Brockington, I. F., Cernick, K. F., Schofield, E. M., Downing, A. R., Francis, A. F., & Keelan, C. (1981). Puerperal psychosis. *Archives of General Psychiatry, 38,* 829–833.

Broderick, P. (2005). Mindfulness and coping with dysphoric mood: Contrasts with rumination and distraction. *Cognitive Therapy and Research, 29,* 501–510.

Butler, A. C., Chapman, J. E., Forman, E. M., & Beckf, A. T. (2006). The empirical status of cognitive-behavioral therapy: a review of meta-analyses. *Clinical Psychology Review, 26,* 17–31.

Chan, S. W., Levy, V., Chung, T. K., & Lee, D. (2002). A qualitative study of the experiences of a group of Hong-Kong Chinese women diagnosed with postnatal depression. *Journal of Advanced Nursing, 39,* 571–579.

Chang. L. (2006). *Wisdom for the soul: Five millennia of prescriptions for spiritual healing.* Gnosophia Publishers.

Chaudron, L. (2003). Postpartum Depression: What pediatricians need to know. *Pediatrics in Review, 24,* 154–161.

Chen, J., Tsuchiya, M., Kawakami, N., & Furukawa, T. A. (2009). Nonfearful vs. fearful panic attacks: A general population study from the National Comorbidity Survey. *Journal of Affective Disorders, 112,* 273–278.

Clark, D. M., Salkovskis, P. M., Öst, L-G., Breitholtz, E., Koehler, K. A., Westling, B. E., et al. (1997). Misinterpretation of body sensations in panic disorder. *Journal of Consulting and Clinical Psychology, 65,* 203–213.

Clay, E. C., & Seehusen, D. A. (2004). A review of postpartum depression for the primary care physician. *Southern Medical Journal, 9,* 157–161.

Codey, M. J. (2009). Hear it from … Mary Jo Codey. Retrieved October 7, 2009, from MedEdPPD.org, www.mededppd.org/mothers/codey_questions.asp.

Cornish, A., McMahon, C., Ungerer, J., Barnett, B., Kowalenko, N., & Tennant, C. (2006). Maternal depression and the experience of parenting in the second postnatal year. *Journal of Reproductive and Infant Psychology, 24,* 121–132.

Corral, M., Kuan, A., & Kostaras, D. (2000). Bright-light therapy's effect on postpartum depression. *American Journal of Psychiatry, 157,* 303–304.

Cox, J. L., Holden, J. M., & Sagovsky, R. (1987). Detection of postnatal depression: Development of the Edinburgh postnatal depression scale. *British Journal of Psychiatry, 150,* 782–786.

Creedy, D. K., Shochet, I. M., & Horsfall, J. (2000). Childbirth and the development of acute trauma symptoms: Incidence and contributing factors. *Birth, 27,* 104–111.

Czarnocka, J., & Slade, P. (2000). Prevalence and predictors of post-traumatic stress symptoms following childbirth. *British Journal of Clinical Psychology, 39,* 35–51.

Dalton, K. (1996). *Depression after childbirth* (3rd ed.). Oxford, UK: Oxford Press University.

Davis, M., Eshelman, E., & McKay, M. (2000). *The relaxation and stress reduction workbook.* Oakland, CA: New Harbinger Publications, Inc.

DeMaat, S., Dekker, J., Schoevers, R., Van Aalst, G., Gijsbers-van Wijk, C., Hendriksen, M., Kool, S.,…DeJonghe, F. (2008). Short psychodynamic supportive psychotherapy, antidepressants, and their combination in the treatment of major depression: A mega-analysis based on three randomized clinical trials. *Depression & Anxiety, 25,* 565–574.

De Montaigne, M. (n.d.). The quotations page. Retrieved January 5, 2010, from www.quotationspage.com/quote/1296.html

DeMoor, M. H. M., Beem, A. L., Stubbe, J. H., Boomsma, D. I., & DeGeus, E. J. C. (2006). Regular exercise, anxiety, depression and personality: A population-based study. *Preventive Medicine, 42,* 273–279.

Dennis, C. L. (2004). Treatment of postpartum depression, part 2: A critical review of non-biological interventions. *Journal of Clinical Psychiatry, 65,* 1252–1265.

Dietz, M., Williams, S., Callaghan, W., Bachman, D., Whitlock, E., & Hornbrook, M. (2007). Clinically identified maternal depression before, during, and after pregnancies ending in live births. *American Journal of Psychiatry, 164,* 1515–1520.

Dugas, M. J., Gagnon, F., Ladouceur, R., & Freeston, M. H. (1998). Generalized anxiety disorder: A preliminary test of a conceptual model. *Behaviour Research and Therapy, 36,* 215–226.

Eberhard-Gran, M., Eskild, A., & Opjordsmoen, S. (2006). Use of psychotropic medications in treating mood disorders during lactation: Practical recommendation. *CNS Drugs, 20,* 187–198.

Edhborg, M., Seimyr, L., Lundh, W. & Widstrom, A. (2000). Fussy child—Difficult parenthood? Comparisons between families with a "depressed" mother and nondepressed mother 2 months postpartum. *Journal of Reproductive and Infant Psychology, 18,* 225–238.

Edwards, E. & Timmons, S. (2005). A qualitative study of stigma among women suffering postnatal illness. *Journal of Mental Health, 14,* 471–482.

Engels, A., Heller, W., Spielberg, J., Warren, S., Sutton, B., Banich, M. & Miller, G. (2010). Co-occurring anxiety influences patterns of brain activity in depression. *Cognitive Affective & Behavioral Neuroscience, 10,* 141–56.

Fairbrother, N., & Woody, S. R. (2007). Fear of childbirth and obstetrical events as predictors of postnatal symptoms of depression and post-traumatic stress disorder. *Journal of Psychosomatic Obstetrics & Gynecology, 28,* 239–242.

Fairbrother, N., & Woody, S. R. (2008). New mothers' thoughts of harm related to the newborn. *Archives of Women's Mental Health, 11,* 221–229.

Freeman, M. P., Davis, M. F., Sinha, P., Wisner, K. L., Hibbeln, J. R., & Gelenberg, A. J. (2008). Omega-3 fatty acids and supportive psychotherapy for perinatal depression: A randomized placebo-controlled study. *Journal of Affective Disorders, 110,* 142–148.

Fry, W. F., Jr. (1992). The physiological effects of humor, mirth, and laughter. *Journal of the American Medical Association, 267,* 1857–1858.

Garcia-Esteve, L., Navarro, P., Ascaso, C., Torres, A., Aguado, J., Gelabert, E., et al. (2008). Family caregiver role and premenstrual syndrome as associated factors for postnatal depression. *Archives of Women's Mental Health, 11,* 193–200.

Gemmill, A. W., Leigh, B., Ericksen, J., & Milgrom, J. (2006). A survey of the clinical acceptability of screening for postnatal depression in depressed and nondepressed women. *Biomedical Central Public Health, 6,* 211.

Geogiopoulos, A., Bryan, T., Wollan, P., & Yawn, B. (2001). Routine screening for postpartum depression. *Journal of Family Practice, 50,* 117–122.

Gjerdingen, D. K., & Yawn, B. P. (2007). Postpartum depression screening: importance, methods, barriers, and recommendations for practice. *Journal of the American Board of Family Medicine, 20,* 280–288.

Goldin, P., Ramel, W., & Gross, J. (2009). Mindfulness meditation: Training and self-referential processing in social anxiety disorder: behavioral and neural effects. *Journal of Cognitive Psychotherapy, 23,* 242–257.

Goodman, S., Broth, M., Hall, C., & Stowe, Z. (2008). Treatment of postpartum depression in mothers: Secondary benefits to the infants. *Mental Health Journal, 29,* 492–513.

Hale, T. W. (2008). *Medications and mother's milk* (13th ed.). Amarillo, TX: Hale Publishing.

Hall, P. L. & Wittkowski, A. (2006). An exploration of negative thoughts as a normal phenomenon after childbirth. *Journal of Midwifery and Women's Health, 51,* 321–330.

Hall-Flavin, D. (2009). *Generalized anxiety disorder.* Mayoclinic.com. Retrieved January 3, 2010, from www.mayoclinic.com/health/coping-with-anxiety/AN01589

Hallowell, E. (1998). *Worry.* New York, NY: Ballantine Books.

Hamilton, B. E., Martin, J. A., & Ventura, S. J. (2009). National vital statistics report, *Births: preliminary data for 2007.* Retrieved November 11, 2009, from www.cdc.gov/nchs/data/nvsr/nvsr56/nvsr56_07.pdf.

Haugen, E. N. (2003). Postpartum anxiety and depression: The contribution of social support. Unpublished master's thesis, University of North Dakota, Grand Forks, ND.

Helgeson, V. S., & Gottlieb, B. H. (2000). Support groups. In S. Cohen, L. G. Underwood, & B. H. Gottlieb (Eds.), *Social support measurement, and intervention: A guide for health and social scientists.* New York, NY: Oxford University Press.

Heneghan, A., Mercer, M., & DeLeone, N. (2004). Will mothers discuss parenting stress and depressive symptoms with their child's pediatrician? *Pediatrics, 113,* 460–467.

Henig, R. (2009). Understanding the anxious mind. *New York Times.* Retrieved November 24, 2009, from www.nytimes.com.

Hettema, J. M., Neale, M. C., & Kendler, K. S. (2001). A review and meta-analysis of the genetic epidemiology of anxiety disorders. *American Journal of Psychiatry, 158,* 1568–1578.

Hipwell, A. E., Murray, L., Ducournau, P., & Stein, A. (2005). The effects of maternal depression and parental conflict on children's peer play. *Child: Care, Health & Development, 31,* 11–23.

Hirai, M., & Clum, G. A. (2006). A meta-analytic study of self-help interventions for anxiety problems. *Behavior Therapy, 37,* 99–111.

Hiscock, H., & Wake, M. (2001). Infant sleep problems and postnatal depression: A community-based study. *Pediatrics, 107,* 1317–1322.

Jacka, F. N., Pasco, J. A., Mykletun, A., Williams, L. J., Hodge, A. M., O'Reilly,…Berk, M. (2010). Association of Western and traditional diets with depression and anxiety in women. *American Journal of Psychiatry, 167,* 305–311.

Jennings, K. D., Ross, S., Popper S., & Elmore, M. (1999). Thoughts of harming infants in depressed and nondepressed mothers. *Journal of Affective Disorders, 54,* 21–28.

Joiner, T. E. (2005). *Why people die by suicide.* Cambridge, MA: Harvard University Press.

Jones, I., & Craddock, N. (2001). Familiarity of the puerperal trigger in bipolar disorder: Results of a family study. *American Journal of Psychiatry, 158,* 913–917.

Jung, C. (1932). John Mark Ministries. Retrieved January 5, 2010, from http://jmm.aaa.net.au/articles/13483.htm.

Kabat-Zinn J. (1990). *Full catastrophe living: Using the wisdom of your body and mind to face stress, pain, and illness.* New York, NY: Delta.

Kabat-Zinn J. (2003). Mindfulness-based interventions in context: Past, present and future. *Clinical Psychology: Science and Practice, 10,* 144–156.

Kabir, K., Sheeder, J., & Kelly, L. S. (2008). Identifying postpartum depression: Are 3 questions as good as 10? *Pediatrics, 122,* 696–702.

Kagan, J., & Snidman, N. (2009). *The long shadow of temperament.* Boston, MA: Harvard University Press.

Kendall, R., Chalmers, J., & Platz, C. (1987). Epidemiology of puerperal psychosis. *British Journal of Psychiatry, 150,* 662–673.

Keogh, E., Ayers, S., & Francis, H. (2002). Does anxiety sensitivity predict post-traumatic stress symptoms following childbirth? A preliminary report. *Cognitive Behaviour Therapy, 31,* 145–155.

Kinnier, R. T., Hofsess, C., Pongratz, R., & Lambert, C. (2009). Attributions and affirmations for overcoming anxiety and depression. *Psychology & Psychotherapy: Theory, Research & Practice, 82,*153–169.

Kleiman, K. (2008). *Therapy and the postpartum woman.* New York, NY: Taylor & Francis Group.

Kleiman, K. R., & Raskin, V. D. (1994). *This isn't what I expected: Overcoming postpartum depression.* New York, NY: Bantam Books.

Knudson-Martin, C., & Silverstein, R (2009). Suffering in silence: A qualitative meta-data-analysis of postpartum depression. *Journal of Martial and Family Therapy, 35,* 145–158.

Kristensen, J. H., Ilett, K. F., Hackett, L. P. Yapp, P., Paech, M., & Begg, E. J. (1999). Distribution and excretion of fluoxetine and norfluoxetine in human milk. *British Journal of Clinical Pharmacology, 48,* 521–527.

Kung, W. W. (2000). The intertwined relationship between depression and marital distress: Elements of marital therapy conducive to effective treatment outcome. *Journal of Marital and Family Therapy, 26,* 51–63.

Lambert, G. W., Reid, C., Kaye, D. M., Jennings, G. L., & Esler, M. D. (2002). Effect of sunlight and season on serotonin turnover in the brain. *Lancet, 360,* 1840–1842.

Larsen, K. E., O'Hara, M. W., Brewer, K. K., & Wenzel, A. (2001). A prospective study of self-efficacy expectancies and labour pain. *Journal of Reproductive and Infant Psychology, 19,* 203–214.

Levinson, D. F. (2006). The genetics of depression: A review. *Biological Psychiatry, 60,* 84–92.

Linehan, M. M. (1993). *Skills-training manual for borderline personality disorder.* New York, NY: Guildford.

Lipsitz, J. D., Gur, M., Miller, N. L., Forand, N., Vermes, D., & Fyer, A. J. (2006). An open pilot study of interpersonal psychotherapy for panic disorder (IPT-PD). *Journal of Nervous and Mental Disease, 194,* 440–445.

Lipsitz, J. D., Gur, M., Vermes, D., Petkova, E., Jianfeng C., Miller, N., Laino, J., Liebowitz, M. R., & Fyer, A. J. (2008). A randomized trial of interpersonal therapy versus supportive therapy for social anxiety disorder. *Depression & Anxiety, 25,* 542–553.

Livio, S. (2007). Promised lifeline for new moms falls short: Postpartum depression law called a disappointment so far. *Star-Ledger.* Retrieved October 3, 2009, from www.netpowwow.com/unite011109/ppdcriminals.htm.

Lockwood, C., Page, T., & Connor-Hiller, F. (2004). Comparing the effectiveness of cognitive behavior therapy using individual or group therapy in the treatment of depression. *International Journal of Evidence-Based Healthcare, 2,* 185–206.

Logsdon, M. C., Birkimer, J. C., & Barbee, A. P. (1997). Social support providers for postpartum women. *Journal of Social Behavior and Personality, 12,* 89–102.

Lyons, S. (1998). A prospective study of posttraumatic stress symptoms 1 month following childbirth in a group of 42 first-time mothers. *Journal of Reproductive and Infant Psychology, 16,* 91–105.

Maes, M., Christophe, A., Delanghe, J., et al. (1999). Lowered omega 3 polyunsaturated fatty acids in serum phospholipids and cholesteryl esters of depressed patients. *Psychiatry Research, 85,* 275–291.

Mancini, F., Carlson, C., & Albers, L. (2007). Use of the postpartum depression screening scale in a collaborative obstetric practice. *Journal of Midwifery Women's Health, 52,* 429–434.

Markowitz, J. C., Manber, R., & Rosen, P. (2008). Therapists' responses to training in brief supportive psychotherapy. *American Journal of Psychotherapy, 62,* 67–81.

Marrs, R. W. (1995). A meta-analysis of bibliotherapy studies. *American Journal of Community Psychology, 23,* 843–870.

Mauthner, N. (2002). *The darkest days of my life: stories of postpartum depression.* Boston, MA: Harvard University Press.

McMahon, C., Barnett, B., Kowalenko, N., & Tennant, C. (2006). Maternal attachment state of mind moderates the impact of postnatal depression on infant attachment. *Journal of Child Psychology & Psychiatry, 47,* 660–669.

McNally, R. M. (1989). Is anxiety sensitivity distinguishable from trait anxiety? A reply to Lilienfeld, Jacob, and Turner (1989). *Journal of Abnormal Psychology, 98,* 193–194.

Meyer, C., & Spinelli, M. G. (2003). Medical and legal dilemmas of postpartum psychiatric disorders. *Infanticide: Psychosocial and legal perspectives on mothers who kill.* Washington, DC: American Psychiatric Publishing, Inc.

Milgrom, J., Negri, L. M., Gemmill, A. W., McNeil, M., & Martin, P. R. (2005). A randomized controlled trial of psychological interventions for postnatal depression. *British Journal of Clinical Psychology, 44,* 529–542.

Miller, P. (2006). Benefits of online chat for single mothers. *Journal of Evidence-Based Social Work, 3,* 167.

Murray, L. (1992). The impact of postnatal depression on infant development. *Journal of Child Psychology & Psychiatry & Allied Disciplines, 33,* 543–561.

Murray, L., & Cooper, P. J. (1996). The impact of postpartum depression on child development. *International Review of Psychiatry, 8,* 55–63.

Najmi, S., Riemann, B. C., & Wegner, D. M. (2009). Managing unwanted intrusive thoughts in obsessive–compulsive disorder: Relative effectiveness of suppression, focused distraction, and acceptance. *Behaviour Research & Therapy, 47,* 494–503.

Nemets, B., Stahl, Z., & Belmaker, R. H. (2002). Addition of omega-3 fatty acid to maintenance medication treatment for recurrent unipolar depressive disorder. *American Journal of Psychiatry, 159,* 477–479.

Newman, M. G., Erickson, T., Przeworski, A., & Dzus, E. (2003). Self-help and minimal-contact therapies for anxiety disorders. Is human contact necessary for therapeutic efficacy? *Journal of Clinical Psychology 59,* 251–274.

Nolen-Hoeksema, S., Morrow, J., & Frederickson, B. L. (1993). Response styles and the duration of episodes of depressed mood. *Journal of Abnormal Psychology, 102,* 20–28.

Nolen-Hoeksema, S., Wisco, B. E., & Lyubomirsky, S. (2008). Rethinking rumination. *Perspectives on Psychological Science, 3,* 400–424.

Nonacs, R. (2006). *A deeper shade of blue.* New York, NY: Simon & Schuster.

O'Hara, M. W. (1995). *Postpartum depression: Causes and consequences.* New York, NY: Springer–Verlag.

O'Hara, M. W., Stuart, S., Gorman, L. L., & Wenzel, A. (2000). Efficacy of interpersonal psychotherapy for postpartum depression. *Archives of General Psychiatry, 57,* 1039–1045.

O'Hara, M. W., & Swain, A. M. (1996). Rates and risk of postpartum depression—A meta-analysis. *International Review of Psychiatry, 8,* 37–55.

Olson, A., Kemper, K., Kelleher, K., Hammond, C., Zuckerman, B., & Dietrich, A. (2002). Primary care pediatricians' roles and perceived responsibilities in the identification and management of maternal depression. *Pediatrics, 110,* 1169–1176.

Oren, D. A., Wisner, K. L., Spinelli, M., Epperson, C. N., Peindl, K. S., Terman, J. S., & Terman, M. (2002). An open trial of morning light therapy for treatment of antepartum depression. *American Journal of Psychiatry, 159,* 666–669.

Papakostas, G. I., Thase, M. E., Fava, M., Nelson, C. J., & Shelton, R. C. (2007). Are antidepressant drugs that combine serotonergic and noradrenergic mechanisms of action more effective than selective serotonin reuptake inhibitors in treating major depressive disorder? A meta-analysis of newer agents. *Biological Psychiatry, 62,* 1217–1227.

Papp, L., Goeke-Morey, M., & Cummings, M. (2007). Linkages between spouses' psychological distress and marital conflict in the home. *Journal of Family Psychology, 21,* 533–537.

Pearlstein, T. B., Zlotnick, C., Battle, C. L., Stuart, S., O'Hara, M. W., Price, A. B., & Grause, M. A. Howard, M. (2006). Patient choice of treatment for postpartum depression: A pilot study. *Archives of Women's Mental Health, 9,* 303–308.

Peet, M., Murphy, B., Shay, J., & Horrobin, D. (1998). Depletion of omega-3 fatty acid levels in red blood cell membranes of depressive patients. *Biological Psychiatry, 43,* 315–319.

Peindl, K., Wisner, K., & Hanusa, B. (2004). Identifying depression in the first postpartum year: Guidelines for screening and referral. *Journal of Affective Disorders, 80,* 37–44.

Pistrang, N., Barker, C., Humphreys, K. (2008). Mutual help groups for mental health problems: A review of effectiveness studies. *American Journal of Community Psychology, 42,* 110–121.

Platz, C., & Kendall, R. E. (1988). A matched-control follow-up and family study of "puerperal" psychosis. *British Journal of Psychiatry, 114,* 37–45.

Raes, F., Hermans, D., Williams, J. M. G., Bijttebier, P., & Eelen, P. (2008). A "triple W" model of rumination on sadness: Why am I feeling sad, what's the meaning of my sadness, and wish I could stop thinking about my sadness (but I can't!). *Cognitive Therapy and Research, 32,* 526–541.

Ragan, K., Stowe, Z. N., & Newport, D. J. (2005). Use of antidepressants and mood stabilizers in breastfeeding women. In L. S. Cohen & R. M. Nonacs (Eds.), *Mood and anxiety disorders during pregnancy and postpartum* (*Review of Psychiatry, 24,*105–144). Washington, DC: American Psychiatric Press.

Rosen, G. M. (1987). Self-help treatment books and the commercialization of psychotherapy. *American Psychologist, 42,* 46–51.

Rosenthal, R. N., Muran, J. C., Pinsker, H., Hellerstein, D., & Winston, A. (1999). Interpersonal change in brief supportive psychotherapy. *Journal of Psychotherapeutic Practice and Research, 8,* 55–63.

Ross, L. E., Sellers, E. M., Gilbert Evans, S. E., & Romach, M. K. (2004). Mood changes during pregnancy and the postpartum period: Development of a biopsychosocial model. *Acta Psychiatrica Scandinavia, 109,* 457–466.

Roux, G., Anderson, C., & Roan, C. (2002). Postpartum depression, marital dsyfunction, and infant outcome: A longitudinal study. *Journal of Perinatal Education, 11,* 25–36.

Rudd, M. D., Berman, A. L., Joiner, T. E. Jr., Nock, M. K., Silverman, M. M., Mandrusiak, M., et al. (2006). Warning signs for suicide: Theory, research, and clinical applications. *Suicide and Life-Threatening Behavior, 36,* 255–262.

Ryding, E. L., Wijma, B., & Wijma, K. (1997). Posttraumatic stress reactions after emergency caesarean section. *Acta Obstetrica et Gynaecologica Scandinavia, 76,* 856–861.

Seehusen, D. A., Baldwin, L. M., Runkle, G. P., & Clark, G. (2005). Are family physicians appropriately screening for postpartum depression? *Journal of American Board Family Medicine, 18,* 104–112.

Sichel, D. A., Cohen, L. S., Rosenbaum, J. F., & Driscoll, J. (1993). Postpartum onset of obsessive compulsive disorder. *Psychosomatics, 34,* 277–279.

Soares, C., & Zitek, B. (2008). Reproductive hormone sensitivity and risk for depression across the female life cycle: A continuum of vulnerability? *Psychiatry & Neuroscience, 33,* 331–343.

STEP-PPD: Support and training to enhance primary care for postpartum depression. Retrieved February 22, 2010, from www.step-ppd.com.

Stone, S. & Menken, A. (Eds.). (2008). *Perinatal and postpartum mood disorders: Perspective and treatment guide for the health care practitioner.* New York, NY: Springer Publishing Company.

Stuart, S., O'Hara, M. W., & Gorman, L. L. (2003). The prevention and psychotherapeutic treatment of postpartum depression. *Archives of Women's Mental Health, 6* (Suppl.), 57–69.

Tolle, E. (1999). *The power of now.* Novato, CA: New World Library.

Tolle, E. (2003). *Stillness speaks.* Novato, CA: New World Library.

Toneatto, T., & Nguyen, L. (2007). Does mindfulness meditation improve anxiety and mood symptoms? A review of the controlled research. *Canada Journal of Psychiatry, 52,* 260–266.

Uguz, F., Akman, C., Kaya, N., & Cilli, A. S. (2007). Postpartum onset obsessive compulsive disorder: Incidence, clinical features, and related factors. *Journal of Clinical Psychiatry, 68,* 132–138.

Warner, J. (2005). *Perfect madness.* New York, NY: Penguin Group.

Wegner, D. M, Schneider, D. J, Carter, S., & White, T. (1987). Paradoxical effects of thought suppression. *Journal of Personality and Social Psychology, 53,* 5–13.

Weissman, M. M., Markowitz, J. C., & Klerman, G. L. (2000). *Comprehensive guide to interpersonal psychotherapy.* New York, NY: Basic Books.

Wenzel, A. (2011). Anxiety disorders in childbearing women: Diagnosis and treatment. Washington, DC: APA Books.

Wenzel, A., Brown, G. K., & Beck, A. T. (2009). *Cognitive therapy for suicidal patients: Scientific and clinical applications.* Washington, DC: APA Books.

Wenzel, A., Haugen, E. N., Jackson, L. C., & Brendle, J. R. (2005). Anxiety disorders at eight weeks postpartum. *Journal of Anxiety Disorders, 19,* 295–311.

Wenzel, A., Haugen, E. N., Jackson, L. C., & Robinson, K. (2003). Prevalence of generalized anxiety at eight weeks postpartum. *Archives of Women's Mental Health, 6,* 42–49.

Wenzlaff, R. M., & Wegner, D. M. (2000). Thought suppression. *Annual Review of Psychology, 51,* 59–91.

Whitton, A., Warner, R., & Appleby, L. (1996). The pathway to care in post-natal depression: Women's attitudes to post-natal depression and its treatment. *British Journal of General Practice, 46,* 427–428.

Wiegartz, P. S., & Gyoerkoe, K. L. (2009). *The pregnancy & postpartum anxiety workbook: Practical skills to help you overcome anxiety, worry, panic attacks, obsessions, and compulsions.* Oakland, CA: New Harbinger.

Winnicott, D. W. (1987). *Babies and their mothers.* Reading, MA: Addison–Wesley Publishing Company, Inc.

Wisner, K. L., Chambers, C. H., & Sit, D. K. (2006). Postpartum depression: A major public health problem. *Journal of the American Medical Association, 296,* 2616–2618.

Wisner, K. L., Peindl, K. S., Gigliotti,T., & Hanusa, B. H. (1999). Obsessions and compulsions in women with postpartum depression. *Journal of Clinical Psychiatry, 60,* 176–180.

Viederman, M. (2008). A model for interpretative supportive dynamic psychotherapy. *Psychiatry: Interpersonal & Biological Processes, 71,* 349–358.

Yonkers, K. A. & Chantilis, S. J. (1995). Recognition of depression in obstetric/gynecoogy practices. *American Journal of Obstetrics and Gynecology, 173,* 632–638.

Zaers, S., Waschke, M., & Ehlert, U. (2008). Depressive symptoms and symptoms of post-traumatic stress disorder in women after childbirth. *Journal of Psychosomatic Obstetrics & Gynecology, 29,* 61–71.

Zane, M. (1984). *Your phobia: Understanding your fears through contextual therapy.* Washington, DC: American Psychiatric Press.

Index

A

Acceptance, 138–139, 208–209
Adaptive awareness, 213–215
Agitation, 63, 75–77, 80, 89, 101, 171
Alcohol use, increase in, 74, 130, 203
Alprazolam, 173
Ambiguity of symptoms, 80–81
Anafranil, 172
Anthropological constructs, 31–32
Antianxiety agents, 173–174
Antidepressants, 56, 89–93, 136, 149, 154, 169–173
Anxiety, 4–17, 27, 61–63, 139, 173–174
    epidemiology of, 5–7
    leading to changes, 5
    responses, 6, 192
Appetite disturbance, 63, 171
Asking for help, 89, 179–181, 186
Ativan, 173
Attachment, 31–33, 44, 212–213
Automatic thoughts, 144–148, 150, 152, 154
Avoidance, 31–32, 47–48, 60, 69–70, 72, 124, 166
Awareness, 98–102

B

Baby, fears regarding
    attachment, 33–34
    avoidance issues, 31–32
    balance, achievement of, 37–38
    bodily sensations, catastrophic
        misinterpretations, 15–17
    consequences of, 31–36
    excessive worry, 9–11
    hurting, thoughts of, 29–31
    impact on children, 35
    impact on marriage, 35–36
    impact on parenting, 34–35
    intrusive memories, 14–15
    nature of scary thoughts, 22–26
    obsessions, 8–17
    obsessive thoughts, 13–14
    perspective, 17–19
    prevalence of scary thoughts, 26–28
    responsibility of caring for, 3–19
    rumination, 11–13
    scary thoughts, as preface to action, 29–36
    thoughts of hurting, 29–31
Balanced response, 149, 152–158
Barriers to relief, 79–95
    ambiguity, 80–81
    critical inner voice, 81–84
    depression, 86–87
    disclosure, 91–94
    half-truths, 87–89
    healthcare providers, 94–95
    propaganda, 87–89
    silence, 80–94
    stigma, 89–91
    support, 89–91
Barsky, Iiyene, 224–225
Behavioral response, 5
Belly breathing, 127
Benzodiazepines, 173–174
Bibliotherapy, 131
Biological vulnerabilities, 199–200
Biology, 39–40, 43–45, 53–55, 86
Biopsychosocial model of scary thoughts, 52–56
Blogs, 134
Blurry vision, 172
Bodily sensations, catastrophic
        misinterpretation of, 15–17
Breaking cycle of scary thoughts, 115–219
Breastfeeding, 53–54, 136, 145, 160, 170–175, 200, 206
Breathing, 13, 15–16, 24, 26, 72, 126–129, 148, 152–154, 156, 158, 202–203
BuSpar, 173
Buspirone, 173–174

C

Caffeine use, 130
Canola oil, 136
Carbohydrates, 130
Caring for newborn, responsibility, 3–19
  anxiety, epidemiology of, 5–7
  bodily sensations, catastrophic
     misinterpretations, 15–17
  distress, 8–17
  excessive worry, 9–11
  inconsistent impulses, 8–17
  intrusive memories, 14–15
  misinterpretation, 8–17
  obsessions, 8–17
  obsessive thoughts, 13–14
  perspective, 17–19
  rumination, 11–13
Catastrophic misinterpretations, 15–16,
     27–28, 50, 54, 71–72, 148, 152,
     194
Celexa, 170
Chat rooms, 134
Chaudron, Linda, 105
Chemical imbalance, 39
Citalopram, 170
Clinical issues, 57–114
Clomipramine, 172
Clonazepam, 173
Coaches, 157
Codey, Mary Jo, 97
Cognitive avoidance, 47
Cognitive behavioral therapy, 143, 161,
    164
Cognitive models, 144
Cognitive self-help strategies, 143,
    146–157
  balanced response, 152–154
  coaches, 157
  coping cards, 155–156
  experiments, 154–155
Colic, 171, 222
Compassion, 31, 104, 112, 158
Complex carbohydrates, 130
Compulsions, 14, 66–67
Computer games, 125
Concentration difficulties, 69, 141, 174
Condemnation, 138

Confrontation, 187–188
Confusion, 76, 183
Constipation, 172
Contamination, 67
Conversational style, psychotherapist, 164
Coping cards, 155–156, 205
Costs of doctor's visit, 132
Counterproductive reactions, 118–123
Counting backward for calming, 125
Critical inner voice, 81–84
Cues from psychotherapist, 164
Cultural mandates, 89
Culture-specific taboos, 90
Cymbalta, 171

D

Dalton, Katherine, 100–101
Dancing, 125
de Montaigne, Michel, 139
Decisionmaking assistance, 164
Demands of motherhood, 18, 179, 211
Denial, 78, 118–120, 123–124, 184
Dependency, 162–163
Depression, 6–10, 32–36, 41–45, 62–66,
    79–81, 100–105, 107–111,
    165–168
  antidepressants, 56, 89–93, 136, 149,
    154, 169–173
  barriers to relief, 86–87
  Edinburgh Postnatal Depression Scale,
    103
  helplessness spiraling into, 32
  major depressive disorder, 63, 65–66
  Melanie Blocker-Stokes Postpartum
    Depression Research and Care
    Act, 103–104, 225
  Postpartum Depression Screening
    Scale, 103
  tricyclic antidepressants, 172
  voice of depression response model,
    162
Depression After Delivery, 221
Depression response model, 162–163
Depressive disorder, 63, 65–66
Despair, 12, 22, 73, 86, 90, 145
Desperation, 75, 88
Desvenlafaxine, 171

Detail-oriented activities, 125
*Diagnostic and Statistical Manual of
   Mental Disorders,* 62
Diaphragm, 16
Diazepam, 173
Disclosure, 84–85, 91–92, 97, 109, 111, 192,
   195, 198–199
Distraction, 118, 124–126, 130, 158, 182,
   202
Distressed thinking patterns, 8–17
Docosahexaenoic acid, 135
Dopamine, 171–172
Dramatic changes in mood, 75
Drug use, 74
Dry mouth, 172
DSM-IV-TR, 62, 66
Duloxetine, 170–171

E

Eating, 34, 77, 83, 203
Edinburgh Postnatal Depression Scale,
   103
Effexor, 171
Ego-dystonic thoughts, 30, 76, 82
Ego strength, 162
Ego-syntonic thoughts, 76
Eicosapentaenoic acid, 135
Empathic statements, psychotherapist's,
   164
Empathy, 95, 104, 112, 161–164, 189–190
Empty words of cheer, avoiding, 186–187
Encouragement from psychotherapist, 164
Energizing activities, 125
Engaged empathy, 163–164
Environmental stressors, 40, 104, 162
Epidemiology, 28
Escitalopram, 170
Essential fatty acids, 135
Estrogen, 44–45
Evaluation of thoughts, 146–154
Evolutionary constructs, 31
Excessive worry, 9, 11, 16–17, 19, 27–28,
   46–48, 61–63, 148, 166, 168, 194
Exercise, 121, 127, 129–130, 147–148,
   154–155, 158, 165, 202–203
Exhilaration, 76, 211
Expectations of cultures, 89–90

Experiments, 154–155
Expression of emotion, assistance with,
   164
   from psychotherapist, 164

F

Facebook, 135
Family members, 7, 41, 53, 75, 174, 181,
   184, 197
Family physician, 108–109
Fatigue, 3, 62–63, 81, 86, 126, 171
Fees for doctor's visit, 132
Fight-or-flight response, 5
Fluoxetine, 170
Fluvoxamine, 170
Food and Drug Administration, 170
Forgiving, 139, 217
Frustration, 51, 144, 216
Future, thoughts about, 25

G

Games, for calming, 125
Gamma-amniobutyric acid, 173
Gastrointestinal problems, 171
Generalized anxiety disorder, 27, 41,
   60–61
Genetic vulnerabilities, 40–43, 56
Group psychotherapy, 75, 168–169
Guilt, 4, 22–23, 34, 63, 65, 83, 146, 181,
   190, 211, 213, 223

H

Half-truths, 87–89
Hallucinations, 77
Headaches, 171
Healthcare providers
   family physician, 108–109
   mental health provider, 109
   midwife, 107–108
   misinterpretation of anxiety, 21
   obstetrician, 107–108
   pediatrician, 105–107
   relationship with, 104–109
Helplessness, 15, 32, 123, 162–163, 218
   spiraling into depression, 32

History of anxiety disorder, 22
Hopelessness, 4, 12, 74
Hormones, 12, 43–45, 51–52, 56, 130
Humor, 217
Hurting baby, thoughts of, 29–31
Hydration, 23, 121, 125, 130, 214, 223
Hypervigilance, 6, 69

I

Identification of thoughts, 146–154
Illness, 67, 76, 87, 89, 107, 181, 221, 225
Images, thoughts in form of, 24–25
Imipramine, 172
Impact on children, 35
Impact on marriage, 35
Impact on parenting, 34
Inability to experience pleasure, 65
Inaccurate beliefs about worry, 46
Inconsistent impulses, 8–17
Indecisiveness, 63
Indicators of anxiety, 50, 69
Indirect scary thoughts, 23
Informational Web sites, 134
Initiative, 47, 108
Injuring baby, thoughts of, 29–31
Inner voice, 1–4, 81–84
Institutionalization, fear of, 83
Insurance, 126, 132, 141
Intentional harm to baby, 3–19
    anxiety, epidemiology of, 5–7
    attachment, 33–34
    avoidance issues, 31–32
    balance, achievement of, 37–38
    bodily sensations, catastrophic
        misinterpretations, 15–17
    consequences of scary thoughts, 31–36
    distress, 8–17
    excessive worry, 9–11
    impact on children, 35
    impact on marriage, 35–36
    impact on parenting, 34–35
    inconsistent impulses, 8–17
    intrusive memories, 14–15
    misinterpretation, 8–17
    nature of scary thoughts, 22–26
    obsessions, 8–17
    obsessive thoughts, 13–14

    perspective, 17–19
    prevalence of scary thoughts, 26–28
    rumination, 11–13
    scary thoughts, as preface to action,
        29–36
    thoughts of hurting, 29–31
Intermittent scary thoughts, 23
Interpersonal psychotherapy, 167–168
Intolerance of uncertainty, 46, 49
Intrusive memories, 14–15, 26–28, 32, 43,
        49–50, 69–71, 83, 194–195
Intrusive thoughts, 8, 14, 22, 48–51, 66,
        185, 223–224
Isolation, 80, 89–90, 95, 101, 133, 191, 216

J

Job stress, 104
Journaling, 131, 201, 204
Joy, 5, 71, 93, 129, 160, 213, 218, 222
Jung, Carl, 138

K

Kabat-Zinn, John, 127–128
Kagan, Jerome, 212
Katherine, 92, 100, 145–146
Kleiman, Karen, 224
Klonopin, 173

L

Lability of mood, 76
Lack of engagement, 63
Lactation groups, 145
Laughter, 130, 203, 217
Lexapro, 170
Libido, 81
Light therapy, 136, 204
LinkedIn, 135
Listening to music, 125, 201
Log, 148–150, 152–155, 158, 204
Lorazepam, 173
Loss of appetite, 171
Lower self-esteem, 83
Luvox, 170

M

Major depressive disorder, 63, 65–66
MAOIs, 172
Marital issues, 104
Marital tension, 36
Mastery, sense of, 218–219
Meaning
    attributed to activities, 124–125
    finding, 217–218
Medical providers, relationship with,
        104–109
    family physician, 108–109
    mental health provider, 109
    midwife, 107–108
    obstetrician, 107–108
    pediatrician, 105–107
Medications, 55, 77, 160–161, 169–174,
        205–207, 222. *See also*
        Pharmacology
    antianxiety agents, 173–174
    antidepressants, 170–172
Meditation, 128–129
Melanie Blocker-Stokes Postpartum
        Depression Research and Care
        Act, 103–104, 225
Memories, 14–15, 19, 26–28, 32, 43, 49–50,
        54, 69–71, 83, 121, 143, 148, 152,
        165, 168, 194–195
Message boards, 134
Midwives, 107–108
Mindfulness, 126–129, 138, 202–203
Misguided interpretation of feelings, 4
Misinterpretations, 8–17, 27–28, 50, 54,
        71–72, 148, 152, 194
Monitors, baby, 155
Monoamine oxidase inhibitors, 172
Moodiness, 12, 81
Morality bias, 48
Mother's Act. *See* Melanie Blocker-
        Stokes Postpartum Depression
        Research and Care Act
Motivation, 47, 111, 190
Muscle relaxation, progressive, 128
Music, 125, 201
MySpace, 135

N

Nausea, 171
Negative social support, 182
Neighbors, 93, 125, 180
Networking, 101, 134, 224
Neurotransmitters, 39, 44–45, 52, 170–173
Newborn, responsibility of caring for,
        3–19
    attachment, 33–34
    avoidance issues, 31–32
    baby, thoughts of hurting, 29–31
    balance, achievement of, 37–38
    bodily sensations, catastrophic
        misinterpretations, 15–17
    consequences of scary thoughts, 31–36
    distress, 8–17
    excessive worry, 9–11
    impact on children, 35
    impact on marriage, 35–36
    impact on parenting, 34–35
    inconsistent impulses, 8–17
    intrusive memories, 14–15
    misinterpretation, 8–17
    nature of scary thoughts, 22–26
    obsessions, 8–17
    obsessive thoughts, 13–14
    perspective, 17–19
    prevalence of scary thoughts, 26–28
    rumination, 11–13
    scary thoughts, as preface to action,
        29–36
Newsgroups, 134
Nonprofessional interventions, 123–136,
        201–204
    breathing, 202–203
    exercise, 203
    laughter, 203
    mindfulness, 202–203
    relaxation, 202–203
    sleep, 203
Nonverbal cues by psychotherapist, 164
Norepinephrine, 170–172
Nurse practitioners, 169
Nurturing, 163, 223

O

Obsessions, 8–17, 26, 60, 66–67
Obsessive compulsive disorder, 26, 60,
    66–68
Obsessive thoughts, 13–14, 26–28, 54,
    65–68, 76, 165, 168, 194–195, 214
Obstetrician, 84, 104, 107–108, 131, 169
Omega-3 fatty acids, 135–136
One-question screen, 104, 112–113
Online support, 88, 102, 134–135, 204
Orgasm, 171
Origins of scary thoughts, 39–56
    biology, 43–45
    biopsychosocial model of scary
        thoughts, 52–56
    catastrophic misinterpretations, 50
    excessive worry, 46–47
    genetics, 40–43
    intrusive memories, 49–50
    obsessive thoughts, 48–49
    rumination, 47–48
    stressors, 50–51
    thinking styles, 45–50
Overly analytical disorder, 22
Oxytocin, 44

P

Panic disorder, 28, 41, 60, 71–72, 92, 167,
    173
Panic-like anxiety, 16
Paroxetine, 170
Passive scary thoughts, 23
Paxil, 170
Pediatrician, 84–85, 105–107, 131
Perception of helplessness, 32
Perception of worthlessness, 63, 65
Perfectionism, 22, 49, 53–54, 179
Personal treatment plan, 191–209
    acceptance, 208–209
    biological vulnerabilities, 199–200
    breathing, 202–203
    cognitive strategies, 204–205
    exercise, 203
    identification, 193–195
    laughter, 203
    mindfulness, 202–203
    pitfalls, avoiding, 201
    psychological vulnerabilities, 200
    relaxation, 202–203
    self-help nonprofessional
        interventions, 201–204
    sleep, 203
    vulnerabilities, 199–201
Pharmacology, 55, 77, 160–161, 169–174,
    205–207, 222
Physician's assistant, 169
Physiological sensations, 50
Points tool for symptoms of anxiety, 139
Postpartum Depression Screening Scale,
    103
Postpartum progress blogs, 134
Postpartum Progress site, 135
Postpartum Stress Center, 10, 83–84,
    98, 107, 109–110, 135, 162–163,
    184–185
    website, 135
Postpartum Support International, 135,
    221, 224
Posttraumatic stress disorder, 60, 68–71
    ideation, suicidal, 73–75
Powerlessness, 137–138
PPD symptoms, 163
Practical support, 91, 178, 181
Praise, from psychotherapist, 164
Preface to action, scary thoughts as, 29–36
Prefrontal cortex, 129
Pregnancy hormones, 45
    estrogen, 45
    progesterone, 45
Premenstrual syndrome, 45
Prevalence of scary thoughts, 5–7, 22,
    26–28, 45, 56
Primary emotional states, 162
Pristiq, 171
Probability bias, 48
Problem orientation, 46–47
Professional treatment, 159–175
    antianxiety agents, 173–174
    antidepressants, 170–172
    cognitive behavioral therapy, 164–167
    conversational style, 164
    cues from psychotherapist, 164
    decision making assistance, 164
    empathic statements, 164

encouragement, 164
expression of emotion, assistance with, 164
group psychotherapy, 168–169
interpersonal psychotherapy, 167–168
medications, 169–174
nonverbal cues, 164
praise from, 164
psychotherapy, 160–169
reassurance, 164
support, 177–184
supportive psychotherapy, 161–164
verbal cues, 164
Progesterone, 44–45
Progressive muscle relaxation, 128
Propaganda, 87–89
Providers, relationship with, 104–109
family physician, 108–109
mental health provider, 109
obstetrician, 107–108
pediatrician, 105–107
Prozac, 170
Psychiatric disorders, 41, 43, 56, 59–60, 166
Psychomotor agitation, 63
Psychosis, 23, 76–77, 82, 185
Psychosocial support, 178
Psychotherapist style, 164
Psychotherapy, 59, 63, 72, 75, 160–169
cognitive behavioral therapy, 164–167
conversational style, 164
cues from psychotherapist, 164
decision making assistance, 164
empathic statements, 164
encouragement, 164
expression of emotion, assistance with, 164
group psychotherapy, 168–169
interpersonal psychotherapy, 167–168
nonverbal cues, 164
praise from, 164
reassurance, 164
supportive psychotherapy, 161–164
verbal cues, 164
Psychotic thoughts, 60, 76–77
PTSD, 68–71, 167
Purpose in life, 75
Puzzles, 125, 201

R

Rage, 74
Rapid heartbeat, 50
Reading aloud, 125
Reassurance, from psychotherapist, 164
Reductions in social support, 47
Relationship with providers, 104–109
family physician, 108–109
mental health provider, 109
midwife, 107–108
pediatrician, 105–107
Relaxation, 126–128, 158, 202–203
Relief barriers, 79–95
ambiguity, 80–81
critical inner voice, 81–84
depression, 86–87
disclosure, 91–94
half-truths, 87–89
healthcare providers, 94–95
propaganda, 87–89
silence, 80–94
stigma, 89–91
support, 89–91
Repeat validation, 113
Requesting help, 178–180
Resiliency, 137, 216–217
Resistance, 78, 88, 94–95, 103–104, 118, 121–122, 131, 134
Response prevention, 165–166
Responsibility of caring for newborn, 3–19
anxiety, epidemiology of, 5–7
attachment, 33–34
avoidance issues, 31–32
baby, thoughts of hurting, 29–31
balance, achievement of, 37–38
bodily sensations, catastrophic misinterpretations, 15–17
consequences of scary thoughts, 31–36
distress, 8–17
excessive worry, 9–11
impact on children, 35
impact on marriage, 35–36
impact on parenting, 34–35
inconsistent impulses, 8–17
intrusive memories, 14–15
misinterpretation, 8–17
nature of scary thoughts, 22–26

examples, 23–26
obsessions, 8–17
obsessive thoughts, 13–14
perspective, 17–19
prevalence of scary thoughts, 26–28
rumination, 11–13
scary thoughts, as preface to action,
  29–36
Restlessness, 6, 74, 126
Rhythmic breathing, 127
Rituals, 32, 67, 89, 166
Rumination, 11–12, 28, 47, 65–66, 83, 146,
  148, 168, 194

S

Sadness, 144–145
Scary Thought Log, 149, 154–155, 158
Scary thoughts, 21–38
  adaptive awareness, 213–215
  attachment, 33–34
  avoidance issues, 31–32
  awareness, 98–102
  balance, 37–38
  biology, 43–45
  biopsychosocial model, 52–56
  breaking cycle, 192–209
  cognitive self-help, 146–157
  consequences of, 31–36
  context, 137–142
  counterproductive reactions, 118–123
  depression, 6–10, 32–36, 41–45,
    62–66, 79–81, 100–105, 107–111,
    165–168
  epidemiology, 5–7
  examples of scary thoughts, 23–26
  family members, 184–190
  following up, 113–114
  in form of ideas, 23
  generalized anxiety disorder, 61–63
  genetics, 40–43
  healthcare provider barriers, 94–95
  hurting baby, 29–31
  impact on children, 35
  impact on marriage, 35–36
  impact on parenting, 34–35
  indirect, 23
  intermittent, 23

interventions, nonprofessional,
  123–136
  mastery, 218–219
  medications, 169–174
  moving forward, 77–78
  nature of, 22–26
  nonprofessional interventions, 123–136
  obsessive compulsive disorder, 66–68
  perspective, 17–19
  posttraumatic stress disorder, 68–71
  as preface to action, 29–36
  prevalence, 26–28
  psychotherapy, 160–169
  routine screening, 102–109
  rumination, 8–17
  screening, 102–109
  self-help strategies, 123–136
  silence, 80–94
  stressors, 50–51
  style, 110–113
  support, 177–184
  thinking, 45–50, 143–146
  treatment, 174–175
  unpredictability of motherhood,
    215–218
Scrapbooking for calming, 125
Screening, 19, 84, 95, 97–114
  awareness, 98–102
  family physician, 108–109
  following up, 113–114
  mental health provider, 109
  midwife, 107–108
  obstetrician, 107–108
  pediatrician, 105–107
  providers, relationship with, 104–109
  style, 110–113
Selective serotonin reuptake inhibitors,
  170
S.E.L.F. care, 129–130
Self-esteem, 83, 142, 160, 162, 216
Self-help interventions, 123–136, 146–157,
  201–204
  acceptance, 138–139
  balanced response, 152–154
  breathing, 126–129, 202–203
  coaches, 157
  controlled breathing, 127–128
  coping cards, 155–156

distraction, 124–126
exercise, 203
experiments, 154–155
identify emotions, 137
journaling, 131
laughter, 203
light therapy, 136
meditation, 128–129
mindfulness, 126–129, 202–203
mindfulness meditation, 128–129
muscle relaxation, progressive, 128
omega-3 fatty acids, 135–136
online support, 134–135
powerlessness acknowledgment,
    137–138
relaxation, 126–129, 202–203
self-help materials, 131–133
six points tool for symptoms of
    anxiety, 139
sleep, 203
support groups, 133–134
thinking, focusing on, 143–146
Self-help materials, 131–133
Self-help strategies, 118, 123, 141, 143, 156,
    159, 175, 201, 205
Self-soothing, 126
Sense of humor, 217
Sense of reality, 76–77
Serotonin, 44, 136, 170–172
Sertraline, 170
Setting limits, 216–217
Sexual dysfunction, 171
Sexual thoughts, 24, 67
Shame, 23, 34, 81–83, 92, 95, 100, 119, 146,
    186, 190–191, 206, 223–224
SIDS, 7, 67
Silence, 80–94
Six points tool for symptoms of anxiety,
    139
Sleep, 61–69, 73, 76, 81, 148, 151, 153–155,
    188, 203, 224
deprivation, 54, 151, 153
disturbances in, 40, 61, 63, 81, 171, 173,
    224
Social networking, 101, 134
Social rituals, 89–90
Social services agencies, 132

Social support, 35, 47, 89, 91, 157, 177–178,
    181–182, 198
negative, 182
Speaking tone, 112
SSRIs, 170
Statement of professional's ability, 112
Stigma, 89–91, 95, 104, 124, 132–133, 206
Stone, Katherine, 92
Stressors, 5, 40, 50–51, 104, 162
Styles of thinking, 45–50
catastrophic misinterpretations, 50
excessive worry, 46–47
intrusive memories, 49–50
obsessive thoughts, 48–49
rumination, 47–48
Suffocation, thoughts of, 67
Suicidal thoughts, 60, 63, 73–75, 112, 188
Superfluous worry, 163
Support, 86, 88–91, 110, 157, 175, 177–184
Support groups, 133–134, 168, 178, 182,
    204
Support network, 181–184
friends, support from, 182
partner, relationship with, 182–184
Supportive psychotherapy, 161–164,
    166–168

T

Taboos, 18, 140
Therapy and Postpartum Woman, 80, 121,
    160, 162, 224
Thinking styles, 40, 45–50, 52, 54–56
catastrophic misinterpretations, 50
excessive worry, 46–47
intrusive memories, 49–50
obsessive thoughts, 48–49
rumination, 47–48
This Isn't What I Expected, 177–178
Thought suppression, 118, 120–121, 123
Tofranil, 172
Tranquility, 129
Tranquilizers, 173
Transitional time, 4
Trapped feeling, 74
Trauma, 14–15, 69–71, 195, 224
Treatment by professionals, 159–175
antianxiety agents, 173–174

antidepressants, 170–172
cognitive behavioral therapy, 164–167
conversational style, 164
cues from psychotherapist, 164
decision making assistance, 164
empathic statements, 164
encouragement, 164
expression of emotion, assistance with, 164
group psychotherapy, 168–169
interpersonal psychotherapy, 167–168
medications, 169–174
nonverbal cues, 164
praise from, 164
psychotherapy, 160–169
reassurance, 164
support, 177–184
supportive psychotherapy, 161–164
verbal cues, 164
Treatment options, 43–44, 51, 79, 87, 89, 95, 125, 127–128
Treatment plans, 191–209
acceptance, 208–209
biological vulnerabilities, 199–200
breathing, 202–203
cognitive strategies, 204–205
exercise, 203
identification, 193–195
laughter, 203
mindfulness, 202–203
pitfalls, avoiding, 201
psychological vulnerabilities, 200
relaxation, 202–203
sleep, 203
steps for breaking cycle, 192–209
vulnerabilities, 199–201
Tricyclic antidepressants, 172
Trouble maintaining accurate sense of reality, 77
Trust instincts, 186
TV, 125, 201–202
Twitter, 135

U

Unacceptable sexual thoughts, 67
Uncertainty, 6, 46–47, 49–50, 146, 153, 190, 211, 213, 215, 217, 219

Unpredictability of motherhood, 215–218
Urinary retention, 171–172

V

Validation, 30, 102, 110, 112–113, 131, 158, 178
Valium, 173
Venlafaxine, 171
Verbal cues of psychotherapist, 164
Voice of depression response model, 162
Vulnerability, 10, 39–40, 42–43, 45–46, 51–56, 139, 175, 184, 189, 201

W

Warner, Judith, 211
Warning signs, 74, 188
Weepiness, 64, 81
Weight changes, 81
Withdraws from others, 74
Wolf, Naomi, *Misconceptions,* 221
Work-related projects, engaging in, 125
Worry
adaptive awareness, 213–215
awareness, 98–102
balance, 37–38
biology, 43–45
biopsychosocial model, 52–56
breaking cycle, 192–209
cognitive self-help, 146–157
context, 137–142
counterproductive reactions, 118–123
depression, 63–66
epidemiology, 5–7
family members, 184–190
following up, 113–114
generalized anxiety disorder, 61–63
genetics, 40–43
healthcare provider barriers, 94–95
interventions, nonprofessional, 123–136
mastery, 218–219
medications, 169–174
moving forward, 77–78
nature of, 22–26
nonprofessional interventions, 123–136
obsessive compulsive disorder, 66–68

perspective, 17–19
postpartum, 63–66
posttraumatic stress disorder, 68–71
as preface to action, 29–36
prevalence of, 26–28
psychotherapy, 160–169
routine screening, 102–109
rumination, 8–17
screening, 102–109
self-help strategies, 123–136
silence, 80–94
stressors, 50–51
style, 110–113
support, 177–184
thinking, 143–146
thinking styles, 45–50
treatment, 174–175

unpredictability of motherhood,
    215–218
Worthlessness, perception of, 63, 65
Writing, 66, 74, 101–102, 125, 131, 157, 171,
    193, 195, 211

X

Xanax, 173

Y

Yawn, B.P., 103, 105

Z

Zoloft, 170